T0150022

STRONGER TOGETHER

My MS Story

CHLOE S. COHEN

STRONGER TOGETHER
My MS Story

Difference Press, Washington, D.C., USA
Copyright © Chloe Cohen, 2019

ISBN: 978-1-68309-236-0

Cover Design: Jennifer Stimson
Editing: Bethany Davis

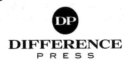

DIFFERENCE
P R E S S

DEDICATION

This book is for my MS family, community, and all caretakers.

ACKNOWLEDGMENTS

To all the people who got me to where I am now:

First I must thank my parents for being my rock through this journey.

Kaylah and Lucas for being my best friends and helping me though all the initial fears and confusion. Thank you for being amazing friends who stuck with me through the initial days and brought me comfort. I thank Laura Widen for showing me the power of positive thinking and helping start the young MS support group. Jim Fairchild for showing me how to be strong and find humor in the face of adversity.

I must also thank the National Multiple Sclerosis Society for all the help and support over the years and their dedication to ending MS.

I am grateful to Oregon Health and Science University for doing so much research to change the lives of MS patients everywhere. Without their dedication to research all that entails MS, we would not be as close as we are to seeing an end of MS.

TABLE OF CONTENTS

FOREWORD

By Marcia Rosenthal Cohen, Chloe's mother

*W*hen asked to write this foreword, I was not sure if the words I would put down could possibly convey the honor in being asked or the emotions involved in capturing twenty-one years of watching Chloe live with multiple sclerosis. But then it has truly been a path that every one of us who know and love Chloe have walked alongside her.

As a family therapist specializing in chronic illnesses, I knew MS from one of my clients. Her diagnosis had been dealt before the advent of all the new drugs, and her life with MS was precarious and painful, filled with hospital stays as she was given steroids. That day, sitting in the neurologist's office and hearing that Chloe's MRI had shown indicators of MS, I felt my blood drain from my body. Not my child. Could not be.

Yet, my husband and I rallied for our daughter and began the search that would lead all of us to a phenomenal doctor in St. Louis and the awareness of three new medications. After a comparison of treatment plans, Chloe went on Avonex. Experimenting on oranges to learn to give shots, my husband was the designated administrator. I think we all cried with that first shot.

Now all of these years later, with fifteen drugs approved by the FDA, treatment of MS has changed. But the walk that each MSer walks still remains a challenge. Recently my husband and I joined Chloe at one of her monthly support group meetings. She and her good friend, Laura, had started this successful group fourteen years earlier. As we went around the room each spoke his or her name, the nature of their MS, and the drug they were on. We were the only family members there that day. I spoke my name and said my daughter had had MS for over twenty years.

Watching Chloe grow and change from a young girl barely out of her teens to the beautiful woman she is today, I marvel at her strength, courage, and resolve. I would be lying if I said it was easy going over the years. Lots of tears, tantrums, depression, demoralizing episodes, and loss. But today as I see this book go to print, listen to her speak at

MS platforms, and head to DC to lobby for change, I think that MS gave Chloe a mission. The MS world is lucky to have her around. Her father, sister, friends, and extended family could not be more proud.

INTRODUCTION

WHY I WROTE THIS BOOK

I wrote this book for all of those people who feel lost and alone when getting diagnosed with a chronic illness. Getting diagnosed with Multiple Sclerosis at the age of twenty, I felt my life was over and that I would never be who I thought I was going to be. Right after a diagnosis, there are so many questions and fears, and I feel like after I was diagnosed it would have been nice to talk with someone else who understood those feelings. I was so grateful to have wonderful, warm, and smart parents who made me feel a little less alone, but because they were not living with MS they couldn't really understand my emotions. I did not know what to do or how my life was going to move forward. The feelings of loneliness and loss were ones no one around me could relate to. Writing this book is one way for me to help others to not feel as alone and scared.

Life with MS is full of ups and downs, and knowing that there are others like you in the world can make dealing with it a little easier. There are so many emotions that arise, and hearing someone else's story can make you understand your life a little more easily. No one has the same path. Especially with MS, no two people are the same, so getting a different perspective on the same illness gives you another way to look at yourself. I am sharing my story with the world to make others appreciate what they have and not what they don't. I am just one of the millions of people who live with MS every day, and each person experiences it differently. Getting an understanding of someone else's experience helps push us further through our battle. Trying to find the right recipe for healing for yourself is key in reaching a place of acceptance and peace. It took me many years to find those tools and I wrote this book to help other people find tools and tricks that will help them in their struggle.

Living a live with a chronic, debilitating illness is never an easy thing, but through the twenty years since my diagnosis, I learned how to navigate in the world and to help others get through the difficulties and uncertainties that this illness brings. Once I was able to accept that this was my life, moving forward wasn't quite as difficult. My path for the last twenty years has been a powerful journey that has taught me how strong my voice is and how I truly do affect people when I speak to them. This path has led me to go from volunteering at the National Multiple Sclerosis Society, to starting a very successful support group, to becoming an ambassador for the National Multiple Sclerosis Society and getting to affect more people. This is why I felt it was my duty to tell my story, to show a positive picture of living with Multiple Sclerosis. All the struggles, all the triumphs, and all the emotions that I went through have brought me to this point in my life where I am actively changing the way people understand MS and bringing about awareness of the massive difference each person with MS experiences. No one can truly know what it is like to live with MS without having it, so I felt it was my duty to paint a picture of my experience and how much all of it made me who I am today.

Hope, strength, and courage will get you to a point where you accept the things you cannot change and change the things that are not helping you live a fulfilling life.

I felt so alone in the beginning and in 2005 I felt like it was super important to start a support group for younger people. Finally, I wouldn't feel as alone and people could come together to share their experiences and be able to hear from others about how they handled a situation or issue. Because the group was geared toward younger people, it was a little different from other support groups because we met at bars and made it a very casual thing.

This group is still meeting, and every month there seems to be a least one new person coming in. Scared to death, they make their way in and sit down with at least five to ten people who know that feeling too well. After the couple of hours amongst others who get it, everyone always leaves with a smile on their face and with more hope in their heart.

They say that sharing is caring, and that couldn't be more true with the MS community. This group has changed my life in so many ways. First, taking the initiative to start the group was scary and challenging, especially because of my physical state. Making it happen was one of the biggest accomplishments I had in life to that point. I have gotten to meet so many different people who live with MS, and no two are the same. Each person has their own disease path, meaning severity of illness, medication, and lifestyle. Together we can help each other through the rough times and exchange some advice on how to deal on a daily basis.

MS doesn't take time off; MS doesn't go away. But when you see your life is not over and that there are many other people out there who can understand, freedom comes.

Every month that I get together with these incredible people, I am enlightened and honored to know how this group has helped them in moving forward in their lives and never feeling alone again. All of us have been there with all the questioning of life and all the fears that arise. These people have become like a second family and together we give each other hope and power to move through life. The love we all share is special and impactful. Being able to celebrate the milestones in each person's MS journey gives all of us power and strength. I cherish my fellow MSers for all the love, strength, and hope we give each other. With time, patience, and determination we can make positive changes and live lives full of opportunity. This path has led me in many directions over the years, but now it has led me to write this book, which I know will help others diagnosed with MS realize they are not alone and that there is a huge community of people who understand their struggles. Together we continue to battle in our daily lives to be reminded of the strength it takes to live with a chronic illness.

Journal Entries: 1999

2/23/99

Today is Sunday, which means it is shot day.

A stressful day. I had a very powerful dream about my shot. All I remember is me screaming and crying about how unfair this is. Why me? Screaming about how I don't want to deal with this anymore. But the whole time I was aware of being out of control and having to deal with the shots. I knew in the dream there was nothing to be done. Very powerful. Plus, I woke up with a cold, which didn't help much.

3/21/99

...There is as much positive energy as negative energy to balance everything. Shit happens, but so do bliss and love. I am positive and have been negative a lot, so I know that when I do find love, the power of that will knock me over. MS, sure it will always be there, but I will survive through happiness. Just when I sit out here, I know there's nothing to stop me from dreaming and loving. I will be a

person with passion and yearning for utopia. Everyone has faults and makes mistakes. We learn from them and change just like every-thing else in nature...

4/16/99

I have been smoking more than usual. Maybe not more, but it is starting to affect me. I need to chill and relax, be productive. I feel so blah and bored, all I know is it is because of the weed. (Not MS). I can not smoke pot. I don't know what I am so freaked out about. (MS maybe?)

9/29/99

I got my shot today around two thirty or so and so I crashed between seven thirty and nine thirty. Now it is ten and I woke up to read some, work, and smoke. My shot really fucks me up, so I'll try and sleep it off tonight. It is strange how it makes my body so sensi-tive and I have to be super gentle. Even fast movement or any kind of lifting make me feels so fragile. Whoa, Ben H.'s girlfriend has MS. He gives her her shot. Strange....

Journal Entries: 2000

12/16/00

When I think of my MS I get scared of the unknown. What is going to happen to me? Will I always be able to function as well as I do now? Why so much anxiety about the shot? Luckily it has gotten better over the year. Hopefully, eventually it will not be a battle in my head every week. Maybe therapy would help. My greatest fear is not being able to predict what will happen in the future. I try to keep the positive attitude, but I still fear the worst. Maybe I will get over this dreaded thing, but the MS is not something you can just get over. I don't think that's a problem. I want to become a stronger person. Move beyond all my issues and get a clear head.

CHAPTER 1

WHO I AM

I was born at the end of October 1977, two and a half months early. I weighed two pounds and four ounces. My lungs were not completely developed. I stayed in the hospital for two months and fought hard to continue to grow. Because I was so small and fragile as a baby, the first three years of my life I was looked over constantly to make sure I was healthy. I was a fighter from the beginning.

I grew up in St. Louis, Missouri, and went to public school. Elementary school went smoothly and I was a very social person. I wanted to be friends with everyone. I was always the one to try and break up fights between people and always tried to be the voice of reason if there was an argument between students. I got in a lot of trouble for talking during class and for distracting people. I wasn't the best student, but I enjoyed the social aspect of school.

I am so lucky to have an amazing, loving family. My father is an amazing architect who had his own firm in St. Louis my whole life. He is an extremely creative man, with a passion for aesthetics and lighting. He is into art and design, so growing up my house looked like a museum. He would rather go to an art museum than any sports game. He was a very creative father who would build the best creations out of cardboard boxes – forts and little houses for us to play in. At some point in middle school we bought a property outside of St. Louis in Dittmer, Missouri. We called it Skullbones Ranch. My father created many trails on this property, but there were a couple that were particularly creative. There was the "Body Parts Trail," which had random body parts all along the path. There were skulls in random places and a severed leg sticking out of the ground. Ten to twenty feet later you would see a pair of hands reaching for the sky. Another trail was the "Nasal Passage." He stuck plastic or rubber noses all on the trees. There was an elephant trunk, a clown, a pig, and even a Groucho Marx nose with glasses and a mustache.

My dad is clearly a fun, youthful man who gives love everywhere he can. He has always been a joker, the prankster, the goofball, and a great soul. His joke-telling skills have gotten worse over the years, but he thinks he is hysterical. That makes me laugh. For my sixteenth birthday, my parents rented a bus to take me and twenty other friends out to the ranch for a scavenger hunt that my father created himself. Everyone wanted to be on my team, but they quickly learned that I knew as much as they did. My team didn't even find our first clue, so we decided to just camp out in the trees and jump out and scare people looking for clues. It was an amazing birthday party that kids talked about throughout high school. Thanks, Dad!

My mother worked as a therapist for near-death and dying patients. She worked with so many people, in so many different situations, and really could change their lives with her words and guidance. She is always there to help anyone who needs it and is one of the best people to talk with when trying to figure out things in your life. She is so loving and caring that as a teenager I greatly disliked her, as most young kids do at that age, but as an adult I cherish every part of her. Because she understands psychology and has a master's degree in social work, she is amazing with people. She does many things to make a difference in the world. She is a wonderful mother, grandmother, wife, and woman.

I have one sister, Erin Daniels, who is five years older than I am, who I was in competition with my entire childhood and youth. She is beautiful and talented in so many ways. She is best known for her role as Dana in Showtime's hit *The L Word*. Her character was very crucial in the LGBTQ community. Erin has done quite a lot of things over the years. I was always so blown away watching her work because she really transforms into the character she is playing. As a kid she would constantly scare me and act like she was possessed by something and would *never* crack a smile. I would be screaming and crying and she would never break character, even at ten years old. I would be screaming, "Erin! Stop it!" With wide open eyes, a creepy gaze, and a low voice, she would say, "Who's Erin?" I would scream and try and hug her and she never broke character. When she wasn't teasing me, we shared the love of music together. Both of us are very musically inclined and one of my favorite things to do was sit at the piano with her and play together. We created a lot of music together and had lots of fun doing it.

I have been an animal lover for as long as I can remember. My family had dogs my whole life. Katie, a springer spaniel, was my first dog when I was a young child, but I do not remember her much. Later, when I was about five, my sister and I were playing outside when a couple drove up and asked us if we knew the puppy they had in the backseat. We did not, but we wanted him. We said, "We will take it and love it." Looking back, I wonder how old those people were and how could they hand over a puppy to two random kids. We took him into the house and made a bed for him out of a cradle I used for my dolls. My parents came home from work and were shocked that we had a puppy, but they instantly fell in love and knew it was time for a new dog for the family. This dog, who we named George, was a purebred Australian Shepard who was more than likely tossed out by a student who wasn't allowed to have a dog in the dorms. At least, that's what I remember my parents saying. George was my best friend and he and I did everything together. He was even known to show up on my elementary school playground looking for me and I would be called out of class to come get him home (we did not live too far from my elementary school). Everyone loved George because George loved everyone. That dog got me through my adolescence when I hated the world and my parents. When I was feeling alone, I had my dog. He always protected me and gave me love and we shared our lives together. We had a pool in our backyard and whenever I would jump off the diving board, George would jump in the pool to "save" me. I loved that dog more than life itself. When George was ten, we got another addition to the family, Sam. Sam was another Aussie because my parents were so in love with George, they wanted another one. I got to go with my mother to the breeder and help pick out the puppy. I wanted a super hyper one but my mother fell in love with another puppy which we named Sam. I didn't care too much and was just excited to have a puppy and fell in love with him. By my junior year in high school, George started losing his faculties. It was sad to watch an old dog struggle, so we had to put him down. I think he was twelve or thirteen.

I was also lucky enough to go to an amazing summer camp for ten years that really developed me into the person I am today. Cheley Colorado Camps taught me strength and persistence. At age nine, I got bucked off a horse and became deathly afraid of those giant beasts. I would not go near one. Before that experience, I loved horses and felt warm near them. One buck and my view of horses greatly shifted to fear. After two summers with no horses, I was persuaded to get back on that horse and beat the fear and really remember how much I loved horses. At Cheley you could get awards or achievements if you studied and did an activity a lot such as hiking, backpacking, riflery, or horseback riding. I studied and learned everything about horses –

breeds, parts of the saddle, what to do if a horse takes off with you on it. My fear lessened and I regained confidence with horses. I became the girl who wanted to ride the rowdy horse rather than running away from them. About three weeks into my second term of summer camp, I received my Horse Patch. This made it official to me that I was a smart, confident rider. Something that I feared so much had become my expertise. This was huge for me. It taught me how to be strong and perceptive. My summer camp taught me so much about life and myself.

At the beginning of the term all the campers would come up with a "code of living." These were qualities of life that we would abide by, and at the end of the term everyone would vote on who best exemplified these qualities. I started there at age eight and spent two years in the youngest unit, and in my final year in the youngest unit I got my "Coup." This was the award at the end of the term that was given to those who best exemplified the code of living. I then moved to the middle age unit of camp and became very involved with horses. After three years in that unit, I received my "Spurs," which was the middle unit's award for following the code of living. It seemed people liked me. I showed all my strengths and weaknesses. I then moved to the senior unit. Those years were the best. I had become a strong rider and had made amazing friends. My final year there I was a junior counselor, which meant I had a little more power with all the campers. That final summer I received my "Golden Key." This was the award for older campers who best represented the code of living. Again, I did it just by being me. This told me that the person I was was one who others liked and wanted to be with. It felt amazing. Cheley showed me if there is a will, there is a way. Every summer they would give out little buttons with phrases on them, sayings like "If it is to be, it is up to me!" These phrases or abbreviations were uttered the whole month. They helped give me confidence and hope.

I was not a big hiker, I was a rider, but I had to do another activity that wasn't riding. I was so scared and unsure if I could do it. I struggled the whole way up and felt like I would never make it to the top. Each step I took felt like I was dragging fifty pounds of rocks up with me. With the encouragement of my counselors and other campers I made it to the top and I had never seen such beauty in my life. When I later got my diagnosis and didn't know what my future held, being scared and unsure, I often reflected upon being on that mountaintop looking over the Rocky Mountains in awe. It gave me strength. The feelings of peace, accomplishment, and relief I felt on that mountain would play a crucial role in how I rolled through the ups and downs of my first five years of living with MS. I can still feel that feeling now. I recall that during one of my first MRIs, sitting in that tube, I reflected upon those feelings I had at Cheley and felt a little more secure.

Another experience at Cheley was my Solo, where campers were put in the woods with limited supplies. I had a tarp, a sleeping bag, two water bottles, an orange, a granola bar, and a journal. It was a big lesson in strength. I did not want to do it. Being in the woods alone for thirty-six hours did not sound like my idea of fun. I was scared to death to be alone, but I forced myself to do it and felt so amazing when I completed it. At the beginning there was some fear, but as time progressed and I got comfortable in my surroundings, I actually enjoyed myself. I spent a long time writing in my journal, braiding flowers into my hair, and carving sticks with my pocket knife. The anticipation of what could happen out there, being alone in the woods, was overwhelming and scary, but what I discovered about myself in that short period of time would play into my life throughout the future. It showed me that I could do anything and that fear is the only thing that holds us back. I took stock in my life at that point and realized how lucky I really was. I reflected upon all the things I love in life, like dogs, braids, flowers, men's bodies. It was another lesson in strength. I was so terrified of what could happen that I forgot to live in the moment. Once I broke free from the fear, I could really enjoy the experience. I remember wandering around the area I was in and coming upon another camper on their solo. I didn't let her know I was there, but just watched her as she sang and danced around carefree with her tarp wrapped around her like a cape. I just observed how much enjoyment she was getting from the little world she created. It made me smile knowing she was experiencing the same joy I was.

Throughout my life, music has been a key for survival. I began learning the piano at age five, taking lessons throughout my youth until middle school, when I started playing the cello at age ten. In fourth grade we got to pick out an instrument to learn. They had all the brass, all the strings, all the woodwinds. Since I was one of the smallest people in my class, someone teased me and said, "I'd like to see Chloe play that big thing." I took it as a dare and began to learn the cello.

During middle school, my love of sound had ripened. I began writing songs on the piano. I played the piano all the time, almost every night after dinner or after school. Once I learned the cello, I began playing it more often than the piano. I had been in the orchestra all through my schooling. At the beginning of high school I really started developing my musical ear and the cello became my biggest outlet for emotion. I could play great pieces already written, but even more powerful was creating my own sound/music on the cello. It enlightened my creativity. If I was sad, I could create sound to capture my feelings. I used the piano to let out my emotions as well. Frustration, confusion, pain, and sadness could get released through the vibrations of sound. As high school progressed, I played more. I went to competitions and had so much fun. I really felt that music was my connection to the world.

Through high school I never had very good grades in math or history, but I had other activities where my skills shone. I was in the orchestra from second grade to my senior year of high school. I was first chair freshman year until a younger prodigy cellist entered my high school. I had also been playing soccer with a group of girls since I was eight. We were a pretty good team and some of our girls were pretty talented.

High school was an amazing time for me. I had many struggles, mostly due to my learning differences. I got extra help. Somehow, I managed to graduate, even though, being the stubborn teenager I was, I refused to do a gym class because I felt like the fact that it required us to tally our activity each week was teaching kids to lie. Nobody really did their required activities, they just said that they did. I am sure that wasn't the school's intention. I know they were trying to get us ready for adulthood, but I really saw no use in this. In retrospect I do think they were getting us ready for the real world in how we did or did not do this, but I was fighting the system and standing up for what I thought was right. I needed that gym credit to graduate, though. I was super fortunate that my best friend's father was one of the coaches and the head gym guy at my high school. He knew I was good with computers, so he asked me to do all of his golf scores and hierarchy for him on the computer. With this credit, I could graduate.

During my junior year of high school I discovered a love for Phish, the jam band. I was blown away by how amazing each musician was and how well they could play music together. They were creative musicians known for their long jam sessions and nonsensical lyrics. My musical listening experience expanded. I liked most music, except thrash metal. Anything that involves screaming, I am not a phan of (pun intended). Phish had generally random lyrics or stories. Their sound was very special to me because of the way they as individuals could play, but together they created magic. I could get lost in the sounds – meanwhile, the lyrics were about the lizards or other nonsense. This was also when my love of reggae music began. I loved the bass in reggae and the messages of love, positivity, and unity with great rhythm. From ages sixteen to nineteen, my life was all about music and the whole hippie culture. I was obsessed. I actually had a dream once about Trey Anastasio, Phish's lead guitarist, saving me from drowning. Yeah, a little obsessed. When I was twenty, my love for Phish declined. I began to get back to my roots of hip-hop and house music.

I ended up going to Fort Lewis College in Durango, Colorado, which is only 111 miles from Telluride, Colorado, where my family had a house. Once I moved to Durango, I felt at home in the mountains. I loved being able to see such beauty walking to class or around campus.

My first roommate in college was an amazing human being and we instantly clicked. She was a singer and played the guitar, which bonded us stronger together. We had so many fun times and on occasion we would play music together. We would go into the stairwell, her with her guitar and me with my cello, and play music to hear it resonate throughout the stairwell. My life at that time was all about music. I started school as a music major because it was my passion and what I really saw myself pursuing.

The first few months of college, I started sleeping through classes and missing a lot of them. I was having a really difficult time with the transition and I was not doing so well mentally. A friend of mine persuaded me to stop taking my anti-anxiety meds because medication wasn't natural. I believed her because I was young and trying to be cool. After I stopped taking my medication, very quickly my anxiety and depression kicked in and I found myself locked in a closet talking to my sister on the phone. My sister came to rescue me and take me away. She flew to Durango and we packed up all my stuff and drove to Telluride. She saved me from this craziness I was feeling. We chilled out in Telluride for a couple days and then headed back to St. Louis in my car. I am eternally grateful for my sister for this because I was really at my wits' end. I always knew that, being my older sister, she always had my back, but this time she really went out of her way to bring me the comfort I needed.

I had to drop out of school at Fort Lewis and move back to St. Louis, which helped me stabilize my life. I had a bunch of friends from high school who were still around, which gave me a social life. I started going to community college that following year, taking different classes to find out more of what I really wanted to study while still studying music.

Spring break came and I decided to go visit a friend in Portland, Oregon. We had so much fun in the week I was there. He took me to the Multnomah Falls and to parks and restaurants and we had a blast. Then I had to leave and go back to St. Louis. On the way into the car to go to the airport, I opened the car door straight into my head. I fell back but just laughed at myself while my friends laughed at me. That bang would change my life forever.

Journal Entries: 2001

7/28/01

Pops has officially passed. The last few days have been extremely long and hot. I've gotten so many compliments. Some people thought I was the actress...wow. This whole experience has brought my family back together. Everyone is so relieved now he is gone. Grammy is doing all right now, but it is going to be hard for her. My family is remarkable. Smoking a bowl on the deck, which my Dad said he designed just for that purpose since no one can see you.

Dr. Cross has told me my options and I am thinking maybe I could do a double dose of Avonex if I could find a nurse to come twice a week to give me my shot. Then I wouldn't be an imposition on Lucas. I know he is happy to do it for me, but I would rather know someone will always be there. At least for the next year, until Rebif comes out. Then I can do the subcutaneous once it's FDA-approved in the US.

8/10/01

I started the double dose of Avonex this week. I think it is fine. I got a nurse to come and do it. She will come to my home twice a week for at least six months or so, depending on when Rebif comes out. So that takes care of that. I did all this shit I needed to do. Good job, Chloe! I should realize that, but really, now what? What happens now?

9/20/01

How can I create music without using an instrument? How can I express myself without music? Will these classes this fall help me find a way? They will at least help me be focused on something other than my MS and my sorrow. I need to snap out of this shit. I realized that I am strong, intelligent, and capable.

Diagnosed with a chronic musical talent.

Ripped of my gift.

Destroying my expression.

Creating an obstacle.

Stuck with a flat without a sharp.

Ivory without Ebony.

*How do I create music without an instru-
ment?*

Poetry and painting?

Sculpture or sex.

The release drives emotions.

*MS pain, sadness, frustration, scary, hope,
fear, darkness, loneliness, fear, codependency, frightened, weak....*

10/18/01

*Today is Thursday, Shot Day. Now I am suf-
fering, kind of. Why do the side effects never
really go away? Should I take more Tylenol? I
guess I am stubborn or it just doesn't bother
me that much. I am stubborn and try to be
tough.*

11/9/01

*There are other ways for me to create music.
I need to get a new mixer for the turntables
and then I will be back in business. I will have
to get a lot of records and milk crates....*

11/12/01

For all the sounds I have created,

I light my torch.

For all who have been ripped of their passion,

I light my torch.

For all those who continue creating sound,

Play on!

It is through you I can feel it again.

And you play music with passion.

I create passion through music.

Now I need to find a new passion.

Where are you?

Please find me as soon as possible.

Journal Entries: 2002

6/4/02

Tomorrow I will see the new neurologist early in the morning which should be OK. I am nervous, but I think it is all good. It's just a reminder that I have an illness more than anything. Then at one thirty I have therapy. Have a lot on my plate right now. I guess just me surviving at this time, although I do need to switch it up so I don't get too bored. I anticipate a really long day tomorrow from seven to ten or something. They'll be cool. I'll be fine after tomorrow – I mean, after the doctor's appointments I'll feel a lot better and even after that therapy will feel better. In between I will go and mail those speakers back to Apple. I'm tired and sick of school, but trying to get by and working hard. I am a Libra. I can do it. It's hard when you're feeling sick and tired....

11/6/02

Harmony. Makes me cry, why? Music, fuck, I want to play music. I'm so sad and angry still. Time is helping me heal that but I'm still sad. I want to create my own sound. The music room is filled with instruments I can't play. I can't create shit. Bob, Ani, Bela, and Victor create such beauty that encompasses so much emotion. I want to let my emotions out to my music, but I'm trapped or some shit. It hurts bad. I can walk, I can talk, but I can't play music. Part of me wishes that my ability to walk was what's more fucked, rather than the arm I use to create music with. The harmony got me, always does. Why can't I get over it? I'm lucky I'm not totally disabled physically but instead I'm musically challenged. Someone come and help find my niche. I need an outlet, bad! Find me? Fuck that. I just haven't found what it is yet. I will. Patience. Fuck! I have to think of something good now.

CHAPTER 2

DIAGNOSIS

*A*fter that one hit on the head from a car door, about thirty minutes into my flight home I noticed my left arm was shaking. It continued to shake, but I assumed it would stop eventually stop. In the meantime, I just sat on my arm or hid it from view. My roommate at the time, who worked in the ER, was very concerned. She knew there was something going on with me that needed to get addressed. She and I went out to dinner with my mother and she asked me to pick up my glass with my left hand to show my mother. I could barely pick up the glass, and it shook in my hand. My mother knew there was something seriously wrong and got me to the doctor as soon as possible. I had no idea what was going on with me, but there had to be an explanation. The testing began. EEG, EKG, and blood tests. All came back normal. The final test was the MRI, which revealed lesions on my brain. "This looks like MS," the neurologist said.

After my diagnosis and seeing images of my brain with lesions all over it, I thought it must have been all that ecstasy I did at parties. I was honest with my neurologist and asked him if this was from the drugs I had done. There must be a reason why this happened to me. He told me no, but I still had a completely different understanding of the brain now. I couldn't take advantage of it anymore with illegal drugs.

The shaking was constant, and I just tried to hide my arm. The vertigo set in about a few weeks after hitting my head. I felt like I was drunk all the time without the benefits or fun parts of alcohol. Shortly thereafter, other symptoms started appearing, like lack of coordination and loss of balance. I was on unstable ground all the time now. I began leaning on walls to walk.

I knew I wasn't going to die, but I didn't know how the quality of my life was going to change. All I knew was that not only did my shaky arm cause problems for my cello and piano playing, but little things like holding a glass became impossible. Without a sense of balance, my hiking and biking days were no longer happening due to a big loss of coordination and balance. Who was I now? All the things that defined me were now impossible to do.

The moment the neurologist said, "You have MS," I had watched my mother's jaw drop and her eyes widen. She had an understanding of what MS was because she had a client who had MS. Her client had been a ballerina, but now was in a wheelchair and could no longer dance. So I am sure my mother thought the worst. I knew that whatever MS was, it wasn't good. My mother is a very smart woman and clearly knew that my life was about to change drastically. Before the actual diagnosis, we had assumed it was either a brain tumor or MS. I was relieved it was not a brain tumor and that I was not going to die, but I was very uncertain what it really meant for my future. I didn't know this disease, but at least there was a reason for everything that was happening to me. I had never heard of MS before. Even though I didn't know what the MS was going to do to me, I was not going to die.

Being that I had been into technology since the beginning of the internet, I got online to see what MS really was and learn as much as I could quickly. The outlook that the internet was bringing me was not very positive. All I saw was sadness and difficulty. I knew that I was not going to die, but who knew if I would end up in a wheelchair. The fear of the unknown was heightened by looking online at information about MS. All I saw online was struggle and challenge.

Back living in St. Louis and trying to be independent and a "normal" twenty-year-old, I went to community college and tried to fit in, trying to ignore the fatigue and learning how to push through. It was rough. During the last few weeks of the semester I got hit with a big spell of fatigue and double vision. I could not finish my classes. That semester was lost and I would later learn that I would not get credit for the classes.

The first few years did involve indulging in alcohol. If I was drunk or had been drinking, I could say it was the alcohol making me uncoordinated and not the MS. Or the alcohol would make me feel better because I didn't have control anymore. It was okay to be clumsy and uncoordinated if I was drinking. I was greatly self-medicating. It was easier to live life in an altered state because I felt so altered without the substances. I felt so lost, angry, and frustrated without them. Eventually, I accepted my reality with the aid of cannabis. But I was so angry that I couldn't take those other risks, mainly MDMA (ecstasy), anymore. I had a totally new view on taking recreational drugs. If I was ever around anyone who was on any mind-altering substance, minus pot or alcohol, it made me sad and mad because I couldn't share in their experience. I remember watching all these people at a party "roll" on X and first I was very jealous and angry. Then, I learned to let it go and was able to watch them enjoy the ride. I could still feel that energy. I could dance to the music and feel it as much as anyone.

Over the years, alcohol was the one escape I really used other than cannabis. Cannabis became just a part of my reality. It was a daily thing that gave me peace with my tremor. The few times I had to go without were rough. I had a battle with my brain. How much of this was extra shaking because I had no THC in my system and how much of it was psychological? Because I knew I didn't have the THC, did it make it worse? Just thinking about my tremor made it worse. I really know how much the mind and body are connected because I felt every emotion through my tremor.

In those initial days of uncertainty and worry, along with all the massive fatigue I didn't eat very much. It took too much energy to make food. Then it took energy to eat. Everything took way more energy than usual and I was sleeping more and more. I lost a bunch of weight, putting me down to ninety pounds. I am barely five feet tall, but this was the least I had weighed throughout adolescence. It was the constant anxiety and fear that took their toll, and I was not eating as much as I used to. I was sleeping constantly and not doing much physical activity.

Day by day I had to learn how to adapt to this world that had no understanding of what I was going through. The physical challenges that I now had to face were rough. I had vertigo. The whole world was unbalanced and on a tilt. I walked against walls or crawled. I was quickly put on medication to stop the vertigo and it went away eventually. My whole left side of my body was now affected. My left side now had a constant tremor that never left. "Are you cold? Do you need a coat?" were common questions I got. Not being able to use my left arm posed a challenge and just made me self-conscious in the world.

Being alone through so much and so many tests led to such uncertainty of my future. Luckily, I had my incredible parents to help me through it all. Having severe fatigue and having vertigo from the MS did not allow me to socialize too much. All my friends were legal to go to bars, but being social with my peers was not happening. My parents were there whenever I needed them. Most of my close friends were in a different space in life. While they got to go around and make mistakes and experience life as an adult, my life was slowed down and I couldn't do what all my friends were doing. I wanted that innocence again.

I wasn't completely alone. I couldn't have been luckier to have the parents I have. They were right there with me through the whole thing. Because my fatigue was so bad, I was sleeping eighteen hours a day and I was only awake for a few hours at a time. My parents were always available for me. They were so under-standing and helpful, even though they couldn't really know what I was experiencing. Dealing with all the changes and challenges I faced in the beginning, my parents never left my side. I had constant ears to listen to my bitching, moaning, complaining, and fears. They never stopped lis-tening. In the meantime, all my friends were working or in school and going about their lives. I felt like I couldn't really bitch too much to them because they wouldn't relate, and I didn't want to burden them with all my negative stuff. This was my battle and I was determined to be the independent woman I had been before. My parents were amazing at giving me the comfort I needed.

I had never considered what a fragile thing the brain was. No one could relate to me. A friend was diagnosed bipolar/psychotic around the same time I was diagnosed with MS. It was a difficult diagnosis for me, but I greatly felt lucky that it wasn't something mental or psychological, just neurological. Sure, my brain was not normal, but at least I could still think straight and form cohesive thoughts. Other than depression and thinking of what could or might happen, I was thinking the same as I did before.

I was going to be independent and in control with my disease. I did not ask for help as much as I needed it. I was stubborn and didn't want to accept the fact that I couldn't do a lot of things the same way anymore. Now I could no longer play music the way I knew, couldn't walk too far, couldn't ride a bike anymore, and I shook all the time. Who was I now? Was I now only defined by my MS? I couldn't be that mountain woman, that free spirited young woman that I was. I couldn't be who I thought I was.

Although when I look back, I think smoking was one way to deal with all the uncertainty that I now faced. Having your life altered so much so quickly was very overwhelming. Smoking a joint definitely calmed my head from the worry and fear of what my future might hold. Not only that, but it made my tremor calmer. I was just a little kid searching for any relief I could get.

As time moved forward, I felt lost and alone. Once self-defined as a musician and an athlete, who was I now? Unable to predict what might come or what else I might lose, I had to redefine myself. I was lost in a sea of uncertainty.

I decided to go back to Durango for school, which made me feel like I was a little bit more independent. I had a mountain man boyfriend who would always help me and remind me of what I did have. The college clinic I was going to for my injections made me feel a little more in control of what I was dealing with.

I always felt so cool mixing up my injection in the waiting room before they would call me back. I think for me it was a kind of in your face, "look what I have to deal with" thing, and it was the only part of the injection process I could do besides get poked.

It was hard to live in the mountains and be unable to do what I once could like bike, hike, and backpack.

But I would always have the stars.

Sometimes my symptoms were visible, but many times not. By observation, most people would say, "I don't see anything wrong" with me. I used a cane more to educate people and let them know I wasn't drunk if I stumbled.

Now I couldn't tie my shoes. All the shoes that I wore were Velcro or I would tie the laces into knots. It was a little frustrating that they didn't make too many stylish Velcro shoes for adults! Luckily, I was not a fan of high heels, but those would not be possible now. That was one of the challenges I faced.

It also took a little longer to do most things. Brushing my teeth, I had to set down the toothbrush then squeeze the toothpaste with the same hand. These little things taught me how to adapt to this new world I was living in. You don't know what you have until you lose it. Anything involving fine motor control was now much more difficult. Moving my musicality to the turntables, there were a lot of wires that connected to the mixer. The grounding wire that attached and screwed tight on the back of the mixer now took so much concentration and effort. I couldn't carry things with my left arm. I could never help clear the table after a meal. Well, I could, but again it took a lot longer. I could no longer cut food. Using knives was not going to happen. Cooking now had to be adapted. As time progressed, I would find tools I could use to help me cook. I often burned myself when attempting to take things out of the oven. I couldn't serve myself salad. When I was eating with people, I could always get help. After some time and more acceptance of asking for help, at a restaurant I would ask them to cut my food for me. If I wasn't with people or at a restaurant, which was most of the time, I wouldn't eat anything I had to cut. I also couldn't type with two hands. I gained some mad skills with the one-handed typing because I was in college.

MS pain, sadness, frustration, scary, hope, fear, blackness, loneliness, fear, codependency, frightened, weak.... I went to Telluride Bluegrass Festival in 2000, and it was a true test of how my MS affected me. Still in denial, I couldn't be that person playing foot bag with all the other hippie kids. The heat killed me. My friends asked me if I wanted to eat and I ending up yelling at my best friends in rage. They told me to calm down and sit down under a tree. Once in the shade I told them I don't know what possessed me to be so mean. I felt the direct change in my body as soon as I stepped out of the heat. My first real experience of the effects of heat and my MS. I was angry that everything was so different now and I couldn't be who I wanted to be. Constantly

I was reminding people how rough life really could be. I always felt like I needed people to be aware of how rough it was for me. No matter what their issue was, it wasn't as bad as what I was dealing with. I later learned that running cold water on my wrists cooled me down faster, which came into play throughout the years.

There was a constant thing in the back of my head saying "You never know what might/could happen," but it got easier to deal with these things. The uncertainty of life would be forever in my head. This would lead me to learn to live in the moment. For ten years, I kept progressing until I started a double dose of Avonex. Avonex is interferon - beta 1a, which was one of the only three medications to slow the progression.

I felt like I was so limited for so long. Being cut off at the bar before even having a drink in my early twenties, that was the worst. Then not being able to stand and mingle wasn't nice either. It would be easier to be in a wheelchair than to be "looking so good." No one could really relate to what I was going through. During college in Portland, I studied speech communications. A few of my speeches were about disability and awareness, but not as much as they should have been. At this time I still wasn't as accepting of my disability or my challenges, but I knew this was something important to show my class. One speech I did was on using the elevator in between classes. There were always a lot of people waiting to get on the elevators and I felt like it was my duty to show them how lucky they were to be able to use the stairs and how they should free space for those who really needed it. I simply made them try to go up and down the stairs on one foot. I made that classroom a little more aware of how grateful they should be for not needing to use an elevator when possible. I was still angry at the world for taking away so much so quickly, but I didn't want to seem desperate or like I was looking for sympathy

I didn't realize the trauma I went through so quickly. I felt raped, but not sexually. Why was everyone so stupid? Why couldn't they understand? I felt so connected to people with disability. I always wanted to help people if I could. I remember one time in between classes when a girl with cerebral palsy asked me to help her with her hairband, but I couldn't do it either. I felt like I related to this woman so much in the short moment we shared. But I also remember that I, too, was disabled like she was. I was trying to ignore the symptoms as much as possible. It was not as easy as I hoped. Trying to be an average twenty-something year old, I tried hard to be like everyone else my age, but they had the freedom to do anything, like go on a hike or bike ride or take recreational drugs.

Reactions people have when I told them I have MS are generally all the same. "I am so sorry to hear that," or "how are you doing?" or "But you look so good." I always say to them everyone goes through their own dramas in life, some are harder than others. In the beginning there were so many things people would tell me I needed to do or change in my life. I needed to start on a vegan diet or go gluten free. I needed to quit smoking. I would also get, "You don't look like you have MS." Nope? I am not in a wheelchair and you can't see my double vision or my fatigue.

Journal Entries: 2003

1/10/03

Head spins and shakes. Alcohol and needles. Worry and relief. Blessing in disguise. A deeper lesson in life, giving me some different edge on life. Pleasure and pain. Happiness and sorrow. Bittersweet...

2/5/03

So, I think I have been fatigued dealing with all the MS having me versus me having MS. I'm tired, bored, and lonely...Self-confidence with my MS....

2/13/03

Watching a video from March 1998, I noticed how coordinated I was and it saddened me. Then I came on playing the cello and that made me even more sad. Right now I just want to escape from this reality for a while, then come back revitalized. I'm feeling completely unmotivated and extremely slow. Maybe it will be better by the end of the week. I just don't feel like doing shit. I do feel like smoking and playing on the computer. I feel stuck with the same old routine, stranded by my own devices. Where, when, and how will it change? I need to make music and feel harmony! I need love and passion....

2/18/03

Took a nap for like an hour and a half when I got back from class but I think it just made me more tired. I'm going to therapy in the morning, which is always good. I didn't go last week because of the doctor's appointment. I do love therapy. It always makes me think and get some insight.

2/19/03

MRI tonight, which is never too much fun. It takes forty-five minutes for the whole procedure. It's not too exciting, but it is very strange. This is the third time I did it, but for some reason this was a bit different. Maybe because I was alone or something. Whatever. Just weird not being able to move and having a jackhammer around your head for forty-five minutes. Wow! Definitely an experience.

4/2/03

I still have double vision. Seems to come and go. I'm totally unmotivated and just keep smoking dope to feel normal. Tired and I don't want to go to school at all. I need to just stop being stubborn or something. Is this MS an excuse? Why can't I just roll with it and have more energy and drive? I'm not feeling it at all. I don't know. It's a combo of hating school and having MS. I don't know what to do. I need to do something besides feel sorry for myself and smoke dope. Fuck me! I don't

know. Skip class tomorrow and sit on my ass all day feeling sorry for myself? Shit! I need a friend to guide me or someone to inspire me. We shall see what happens. Please, something happen in my life that's more positive!
Any day now. Can't take it anymore!

4/13/03

Still feel a bit discombobulated. I don't know what is going on with me. I don't know if it's MS-related or normal or what. I'm bored and tired. I don't want to take this fucking web class but I need one more class in the summer. If I just force myself and stop the bullshit.... I need something exciting to happen in my life. Something that is worthwhile.

It turned out that after I broke up with my boyfriend, I realized I didn't know anyone and thought maybe I should move somewhere else. That is when I decided to move to Portland in the summer of 2000.

Journal Entries: 2005

9/22/05

Throughout the years of living with MS, I have gained a perspective that most don't get until late adulthood. Well, I got it at a young age. At first I was angry at every able body around me. Why did I have to deal with life like this? Why couldn't the able-bodied people deal with something like this? I will use this strength. Now. I will use this to empower me. Because I endure this, I gain more strength. It is OK to complain. Please allow bitching. There is never an escape. There is no way to forget or act like MS doesn't exist. For me, I feel constantly reminded of my ailment. I will find distractions and I do find distractions, but they are only temporary. There is no true escape ever. I distract or I deal with marijuana. Is it a distraction from the constant annoyance or is it an aid in how to deal with a constant annoyance? How do you handle something that is annoying to deal with? So I smoke pot. I spin records. I get on the computer. I can't stop and feel normal ever again. Will this become "normal"?

Is it a curse to have such an ailment or is it a blessing to have this perspective? Do I want to go frolic on the beach? How do I deal with such losses? I try and move on, but this ailment will always hold me back. Is attitude everything? Yes, but it will not cure us, but it keeps us healthier. How you think affects how you feel physically. You think, therefore you are.

Unpredictability is difficult to live with. There is always the possibility and chance, but by taking care of yourself you lower those chances. No longer being able to do shit you could once do sucks! But you learn to do new and different things. I guess, I will constantly be doing different things. I hope so. I really don't know how to recover, but it is possible. We bounce back, we adapt, and we try to move on. Time passes and we heal. Time is the best healer. It is just a bit more intense when you are so young. Growing into an adult and becoming my own with this ailment is unique. Discovering adult life as someone who deals.

10/9/05

Tonight was the dinner of champions honoring Grammy for the NMSS. I spoke *at it and totally shocked myself. In a sense I greatly touched the whole room. So many different people came up to me and told me how touched they were. I know I am good at this. I know I made a huge impact on all of the hundreds of people there tonight. Wow! It feels incredible to speak so well and affect so many people. I feel so blessed/grateful. I got a freaking standing ovation. This was so spectacular for the MS Society. I know I raised at least $50,000 for research. At least fifty people came up to me and told me how I touched them. It feels good that people heard me and got a glimpse through my lens. Is MS the center of my life? Yes, and no. I feel like my life is run by medicine. Avonex, Lexapro, anti-fatigue meds. Will it always be? I hope not. I guess my life is driven by the MS. Everything I do revolves around my MS. It is time for more in life....*

CHAPTER 3

TREATMENT

J began treatment, Avonex, in 1998, a couple months after my actual diagnosis. At this time there were only three drugs to slow the progression of the illness. These were called the ABC drugs: Avonex, Betaceron, and Copaxone. All three were injectables. This presented a whole new challenge on top of all the physical ones. I don't do needles. What do you mean I have to get injected once a week for life? There is no pill I can take. The anxiety that welled up every Sunday when I had my father do my injection was not fun. I learned tricks to get through this weekly anxiety attack as time progressed. The first trick was to have my mother on one side of me talking about something so that my attention was distracted and my father would do the dirty work on my other side. The second trick was wiggling my toes on the opposite side of the injection, which I learned in Colorado from a nurse at school. Once, in Oregon, my amazing therapist helped me learn how to visualize. I would visualize a bright red ball and watch it float away in my head. Once it floated away, the injection was over.

Injections make life very real. I was hyper-aware of the moment. I was one of those kids who ran from the doctor when it was shot time. I always hated needles. Because I had a fear of needles I was never able to do my own shot. For fifteen years, someone else did my injection. A year ago, I started using the Avonex Pen, and it changed my life completely. Even now, after using the Pen for over a year, there is still a moment of panic before I push the button. I think there was so much anxiety for me in those beginning years that even now that I have been doing it for so long, on occasion that anxiety comes up. The initial days of all-day anxiety prior to an injection were the worst. My two best friends used to take a shot of vodka when I would have to get my injection. I didn't take the shot of vodka, but I did get a dose of Avonex. They made "shot time" a little easier. I always rewarded myself with cannabis after the shot was done. Cannabis was the only thing that gave me relief from my tremor and the side effects.

Side effects of the Avonex were dreadful for the first few years. Three extra strength Tylenol before injection and usually two or three more about five hours after the injection

Once I was in Oregon, I continued my college experience at PSU. I went to the clinic at the school. At this point I had to move my injection site from the top of my thighs to my hips. My legs had started developing scar tissue, so I moved to the hips because it was the most fatty and not in my visual field. The nurse at the PSU clinic was the one who taught me to wiggle the toes on my non-needle side while getting my shot. This focused my brain on the other side of my body and less on the needle side. All the nurses at PSU were kind in helping me with making my shots as easy as possible for me.

At twenty-two, I had my second episode of double vision. It was worse than being drunk because you view the world like you're drunk, but you didn't have the fun part of intoxication. The double vision lasted a couple of weeks until I was able to get some steroids to calm the flare. It was really hard to be in school while this was happening. Because of these episodes, it took me a few years longer to graduate college.

I was quiet about my MS with my professors at first, but after missing so many classes I became vocal with them about the MS. I then got more help and more understanding about the challenges of school and dealing with MS on a daily basis. At twenty-four and again at twenty-six, I had bouts of double vision and more steroids. Because of these three episodes of double vision, if I were to have more than one drink of alcohol, I would be seeing double. Eye patches made it easier to see if I was going to have more than one drink.

It was a major perk to now be in Oregon where I could legally use my other medicine, cannabis, and get relief legally. Not only did it bring me physical relief, but also psychological relief from having to live with a chronic illness and all the what-ifs of living with MS. As someone who had smoked before my diagnosis, I knew the feeling, but my MS diagnosis took my relationship to cannabis to a whole new level and understanding. Now, I wanted everyone to understand the power of this plant. I became involved with medical marijuana groups in the city. There were many people who understood the power of this healing plant as medicine. I met so many people with so many different ailments. Even with chronic pain, HIV, or tremors, all could find some relief without the need for as many pharmaceuticals. I met all kinds of people who truly understood the power of this medicine. People studied the power and were scientists about cannabis. I feel lucky to have lived in such a great place with these understanding and knowledge-seeking people.

I became eligible for medically legal cannabis in 2004. I was lucky to live in a state where it has been legal medicinally since 1998. I was able to grow my own medicine so I knew what was in it, how it was grown, and could choose strains that were most effective for my issues.

Growing cannabis is a full-time job that requires a lot of time, patience, and energy to create quality medication. I grew my own for many years. When I started growing, I was unable to keep up with the watering due to lack of energy and coordination. I adapted my grow to me. At first, I had a buddy help me grow by coming by every week to check on my plants. It was extremely helpful to have another set of eyes on my girls. I eventually got a self-watering system to make it easier for me to keep up with the watering and not having to lug out gallons of water myself. Because my coordination wasn't the best, this system made it easier for me to keep the plants healthy and happy. Learning how to adapt my grow to work for me was the best move I made.

For a couple of years I used this system until I felt confident enough in my body. I stopped using the autowatering system and began hand watering my plants. I spent around thirty minutes to two hours a day checking on my plants. The process of growing is time consuming and super rewarding. All the energy and time I put into the plants would give me incredible medicine that kept me functioning to the best of my ability.

Creating life from a seed that needs to be cared for and monitored constantly to become a beautiful, potent medicine is quite the process to watch. It definitely takes a while, a few harvests, before you become really dial in and can get the best quality out of your grow. There is a lot of frustration discovering what works and what doesn't. There are a few times that your grow doesn't come out successful, but after some time and some fails, the end result is bountiful. I babied my seedlings and made sure I gave them all the love they needed to grow into beautiful plants. My indoor garden sat behind a wall behind where my turntables were in my basement and I knew that the plants craved music. I think they enjoy the vibrations. I played music on one side of the wall while my plants grew majestically in their room.

Once cannabis became recreationally legal, my growing slowed down because I had access to so many different strains at many different dispensaries. I was a card holder, which allowed me to not have to pay taxes on my medicine.

Also, card holders get priority in dispensaries, allowing us to go ahead of those without cards. Because there were so many dispensaries around me, I rarely had to look too far for what I wanted. I miss growing and will probably start up again once I have the time to commit to it. There is such a rush knowing that after months of growing you can finally harvest your crops, wait a bit for them to dry, and then really relish in what you have created. I often had people over to help me trim due to the lack of coordination with my left arm. Luckily, there are always people who enjoy helping out in this phase. The results of all that energy and effort payed off in full when I was able to look at the many jars on the table full of fresh, potent medicine that I could use at my leisure.

Before it was recreationally legal it was a lot easier to have access to clones, seeds, and plants through other medicinal card holders. Now, there is not as much community for medical patients as there once was.

When I was diagnosed, all I wanted was a pill instead of an injectable. Now there are pills, infusions, and – still – needles. The advances they have made in medications blows me away. I never thought I would get used to getting injections. Since I've been doing double dose

Avonex, I have not had any flares or relapses for many years, but I was still unable to do my own injection for fourteen years.

As time moved forward, I felt lost and alone. Once self-defined as a musician and an athlete, who I was was lost in a sea of uncertainty. I began treatment, Avonex, a little while after my actual diagnosis. Cannabis gave me relief of the side effects of the medication, which for me was major muscle tension in my legs and extreme nerve sensitivity. I remember crawling into bed and feeling like the sheets were sand-paper scraping my legs. This slowly lessened over time.

As time progressed the anger and fear lessened. There is forever a constant voice in the back of my head saying, "You never know what might/could happen." This led me to learn to live in the moment. For ten years, I kept pro-gressing until I started a double dose of Avonex.

Who knew I would get used to needles. Since I've been doing double dose Avonex, I have been in remission, no new episodes, yet I was unable to do my own injection for fourteen years. Then the Avonex autoinjector came out and I knew after fourteen years I could do my own injection finally. It was simple. I knew what it felt like to get an injection, yet these needles were way smaller than those I used for so many years. The nurse came to my house and taught me how to do it and I got to practice on a fake skin surface. It was the simplest thing and there was very little anxiety. Pushing that little button does create a lot of anxiety, but it's quick and fast and now it's only a passing thought. I do believe it's been over two years and my life has changed completely by not having to worry about going somewhere to get my injection done. I do miss the clinic for the warmth and social atmosphere it brought. Because it was such a big part of my life for so many years I had a closeness to all the staff there. In the last couple years, going back just for a regular doctor's visit always feels awesome.

Journal Entries: 2006

1/12/06

My tremor took away my ability to play certain instruments. The piano and the cello. The instruments I was pretty darn good at. It limits me. I'm self-conscious about it. I always think people may wonder the wrong thing. I don't want to explain, but feel as if it is my duty. Really I know people aren't looking at me wondering. Even though I know this, I'm still super self-conscious. I feel like there is so much to deal with if I let someone in that close. I hide it and I get frustrated. I hate that I cannot get a task done with my left arm, simple things like holding a glass. Washing my face with two hands took many years of practice. If this illness had to take something, why my arm? The grass is always greener. Why music? Damn! This is my life challenge. Who would I be without MS? Weird. How would life be so different? Will this tremor always make me self-conscious?

The Terrible Tremor

Stop Shaking.

It will go away.

Difficult

It's gonna be OK.

Abnormal

Fuck.

Not fair.

Frustration

Bitterness

1/17/06

Why my arm? Why my legs? Why my eyes?

It drives me crazy. Wanted it to be controlled. Want to control it, but can't. So angry that my music was taken, stolen, ripped from me. So angry that everything is a little bit more challenging for me. I so hate that every intense emotion is felt in my body outwardly. I hate that my body gives away my mind. So I don't put myself in those situations where my body would be showing it. I just wish it was different. I wonder if acupuncture could stop my tremor? Who am I without this tremor? If it stopped, I would want to play music again but would have to start at the beginning.

7/16/06

Life's been slow due to a bout of fatigue that lasted about three weeks and it sucked. It finally dissipated yesterday. I couldn't do anything, but I try. So I'm officially smoking again. It actually got me out of the house.

Journal Entries: 2007

11/30/07

Fatigue is not fun! Thought it was gone, but no. Taking meds for it now. No longer being stubborn. Fuck that adolescent behavior about that shit.

12/14/07

This damn fatigue sucks and I can't seem to shake it. My life is pretty slow right now. I sleep and yawn. I don't even get stoned right now. I am in a slump and hope it turns around soon. I have no true excitement going on right now. I am feeling stuck. I don't know how to get up again. I haven't spun records in a few days, so I know it's bad. But I also know it will get better. I really need to meet some new people and get out there somehow. I am not too sure how. I will never find a man or even friends if I don't leave the house. I feel bad for Hatchet because I am so tired. I can't take him places because I don't go anywhere. I guess I am kinda depressed, but won't admit it. I just feel like I can't do anything. I have no motivation to try and make anything happen at this point. I miss Mr. DJ. I miss the reminder of how hot and sexy I am. It feels good when someone really likes you. It has been so long since I have had a real relationship and I miss it. I miss feeling needed and wanted. I miss needing and wanting someone. This is why I am missing him. It's not him, but how he made me feel. Man, I wish life was different. I wish I didn't spend my life at home and alone. I really need a change. I need a new person in my life. I guess now is not the time. Hopefully this fatigue will lift and I can try to actually be productive about myself. One day things will change.

CHAPTER 4

RECLAIMING MY HEART

*I*n 1997 I started using a computer program called iVisit, which was a video chat social platform where people from all over the world could connect. It really became my main source of social interaction. I didn't use it much in 1997, but once I was diagnosed it became my one social outlet. On this program no one could see my physical limitations very clearly and it really made me feel like I had a normal social life. Because my fatigue was so bad and I was sleeping eighteen hours a day, I would use my waking time to talk to others. It kept me social and I became very close to a lot of these people, who seemed to mostly live in Europe. We spent almost every day talking to one another. I talked with a few people from the Netherlands on a daily basis and greatly wanted to visit them. The one major problem was how I was going to get my injections done if I went there. I was lucky because my Dutch friends said it should not be a problem to go to a clinic and get it done.

This was great news and I told them it would happen at some point.

I used iVisit until 2009, when it officially died. At that point I discovered Google+, which gave me a new social community and a new avenue to DJ for new people. In the beginning of Google+ Hangouts, I had a weekly show that brought in a lot of viewers. Eventually, the show I was a part of died, and I would just open my own hangout and see who came in. It was always an adventure. I sometimes took requests, but generally I just played what I wanted on the fly. This new program allowed me to meet people from all over the world and became my new iVisit, where I could DJ for people and socialize.

Finally, in 2006, I visited Holland for the first time. It was amazing because I got to finally meet twenty-one of my European friends from online. It was a great trip, but I felt more disabled and had to adapt much of my activity. Because the streets are mostly cobblestone, I could not look up at what was around me unless I stopped. The place I was supposed to stay in was not handicap accessible, which made it very difficult for me. Luckily, my Dutch friends rescued me and I stayed with them, which was all flat, no stairs, and more comfortable. I loved going to the clinic there to get my shot done. I just walked on in and sat for a few minutes and they called me back and the shot was done. So simple and so easy. It was the first time I had traveled by myself across the ocean and was independent. No service dog to clue in people, so I took my cane. It helped me not feel so self-conscious about my "drunk walk." I fell in love with the Netherlands.

The best was going to the clinic to get my injection. One of my favorite things was that I could be smoking a joint as I walked to the clinic. I could set it down, go in to do my injection, which took like ten minutes. I stepped out of the clinic and could pick up my joint and continue to smoke it right after I got poked. What a freedom.

Cannabis had given me relief from all the physical symptoms, but even better was the psychological relief. I went to a coffee shop with my friend. Being that I was medicinally legal in Oregon, I had gained a lot of knowledge on cannabis. When looking at a menu in the shop, I picked out one of the stronger strains. The bud tender looked at me, because I was American and said in Dutch, "This might be too much for her." My friend, in Dutch, told him I knew my cannabis, was legal in the states, and had MS. The bud tender said in Dutch, "OK, I will give her what she wants." Without my Dutch friend being with me, it would have never happened. I was in love with this place where I could use my medication freely and no one second-guessed why.

In 2008, I went back to Holland to hang out with the wonderful people again. This time I stayed in a hotel, which was very convenient. I took cabs rather than walking and honored my body by not pushing too hard and maintaining a calm, accessible, and safe trip. I still could not look up unless I was not moving. My friend wanted to take me to a coffee shop on a boat, but my body wouldn't allow it. The rocking of the boat was making me dizzy and unbalanced. I was disappointed, but we just went to a different coffee shop. This trip let me be independent, with the help of my Dutch friends. I got to spend the days with my new Dutch family. We had many good times and one day my friend Patricia and I went to Amsterdam for the day and got to peruse the streets with all their history and beauty. We went to a couple of coffee shops and walked through the red-light district. My friend had to use the bathroom, so we quickly walked through; I didn't see too much. I saw a few girls in windows, but I was looking down most of the time so I did not fall. Once we returned back to my friends' home, I was asked what I thought of the red-light district and I said, "Not too much because I wasn't really looking around much. Just determined to find a bathroom." And at that point I kind of considered Amsterdam to be the dumpster of the Netherlands. So much beauty and history that was smothered in homelessness and junkies. I knew, though, that I would be back again when I really could explore more.

I went back to Holland in 2010 and my Dutch love continued. This time I did it the best by renting an apartment that was modern, colorful, and perfect for me. I slept a lot, mostly because of all the walking on cobblestone. I am so thankful that I was able to walk as much as I have. It is hard. I do work out for hour-long sessions with my trainer, but during that hour I am doing so many different exercises that it doesn't seem as exhausting. I think just walking can be too challenging for my brain. I have to keep switching it up and activating different parts of my brain and not just the walking part. I am so lucky to know how my body works and how to respect what I have. I am so honored to have this life and know what it is like not to be able to do so much and now being able to do so much more. I keep getting better and healing myself.

The Dutch have an incredible way of looking at disability. They don't see it like Americans do. There was not a stigma around me because I was using a cane. In the US, I got looks and stares. The view of disability was vastly different from the US. The second time I came with my cane and was walking along, I spoke to a woman on the street and she asked me if I was hurt and I told her no, that I had MS. She then proceeded to tell me she knew what MS was and many people in Holland suffer as well. I noticed quickly how the awareness of disability was much higher there. They did not see disability as a flaw like most Americans. Another Dutch man I met said to me, "So, you have MS. My eyes are blue and your eyes are brown," we all are different and go through our own struggles. MS does not define me.

Everyone bikes in Holland, but there are so many people on scooters. I never had to use a scooter, but I think it would/could be a very nice thing. The Dutch are such kind, positive people. It isn't about the quantity, but the quality. It was such a nice thing to be able to get out of my little bubble of Portland and travel across the ocean and see another culture, another way of life. I wish more Americans were able to get out of their bubbles and see the diversity of the world. I loved seeing different, new ways of doing the same things or new things. I am so lucky to know how much is out there and be able to travel and see more than most.

In 2015, I returned to Holland to hang out with one of my favorite people I had met online back in 1998 who was a special friend, more like family. After knowing each other for so many years, he had watched my battle with MS over the years and was so impressed with my walking and energy. He took me all over Eindhoven and showed me so much about his life. I got to see where he went to school, where he had worked, and I got to meet his family. It was so special to be there with him and meet the people who created him. He took me on a short hike around a lake where he spent a lot of time during his youth. It was so special to share this time with him and have the energy to do all that I did with him. He was very kind and curious about making sure I was doing okay and sat down enough. I think I got him addicted to coffee that trip. Being the coffee junky that I was, I shared the joy of good coffee with him and he hasn't looked back. He is totally a coffee junkie now. Thank you, coffee, for getting me through so much fatigue and brain fog! Coffee will always be a drug of choice for me and I will love my morning coffee for the rest of my life.

Most recently, I got to go back to Amsterdam with my friend from England who came to visit me while I was there. I could finally experience Amsterdam with my eyes looking up. We went to a couple of museums and coffee shops. I was in another place where my confidence had risen and my options were open. This was a special trip.

In 2007 I was in a horrible car accident. This accident happened because of my tremor and me thinking I could grab a drink with my right hand in the center console. While holding on to the wheel with my left hand, it decided to jerk while I was going sixty mph. I was in shock, getting pulled out of the car through the window. My first question was, "Where are my dogs?" who were in the car. Someone told me they saw them jump out of the car. Not concerned about myself, all I could think of was my fur babies. Because I was in shock, my legs were not working so well and walking to the ambulance I was held up by the EMT. I didn't feel hurt, my passenger wasn't hurt, but my dogs were gone. I told the EMT I had MS, which explained my difficulty walking.

I could really never trust my body anymore. I was now scared to death of driving because I never knew how my body was going to act. The trauma of the accident and losing my dogs lingered with me for a very long time, but through hard work and many tears I found peace with the loss of my cello, which had also been in the car. It became more about the trauma of my diagnosis than the trauma of the car accident.

After being in this horrible car accident, I suffered from a little PTSD and was very scared when driving. I didn't drive for a year because of this fear. I slowly regained a little more confidence when driving. Because my accident was caused by my tremor, I had so much distrust of my body. It was hard to accept this, but I would continue to work on it. I will always have a little anger, sadness, and frustration about not having control over my body anymore.

Through lots of talk therapy and eye movement desensitization and reprocessing (EMDR) therapy the fear lessened, and my new job was now to learn how to adapt in the world. EMDR was the most intense process of therapy I had ever done. It was also the most difficult and painful therapy I had done. But, only through that pain could I find healing through my trauma. It brought me to a new place of acceptance and understanding.

I had to get animals back in my life. Those first couple of weeks with no animals at home were brutal. My whole life I'd had dogs and not having one in my home was very strange and way too quiet. I went and got two kittens right away so I could have the animal love quickly. I looked for a new dog, but couldn't find one at the pound. I went and bought a pug puppy for the instant love and cuteness. My new little dog gave me the dog love that I needed. He was the cutest puppy and brought smiles to everyone who met him. After a bit of time I felt like maybe I should get a service dog because I didn't know what this disease was going to do to me in the future. I found a woman on MySpace who trained dogs to be service animals for whatever need. I told her about my MS and how I was really wanting a dog for mobility.

This soon-to-be fur baby was trained for a year specifically for me. I flew to pick him up in Indiana, where I would meet the whole litter of pups. His name was Hatchet and he was to become my best buddy. He would give me security in the world. Having a dog by my side at all times to help me navigate through the world made being in public easier.

I am definitely more of a dog lover then anything, so not letting people pet him was difficult. I eventually got a patch for his vest that said, "Working dog. Please ask to pet." I understand why service animals should not be distracted while working, but I felt that Hatchet was there for me not only physically, but emotionally. I would tell people every time they asked to pet him that most service dogs should not be petted or distracted from their job, but I was so grateful and lucky to have such a smart, amazing dog who I wanted to kind of show off to the world. Hatchet was my right-hand man and let me feel more comfortable out in public.

Journal Entries: 2008

2/26/08

I am trying to read more because I feel the MS stole a lot of my reading abilities. My neurologist said that I just don't read enough. I tell her the difficulties I have with reading and she says practice, so I am trying to read more. I started Harry Potter again last week and I can tell that it is getting a little easier. Before, I had to read the same line at least three times before I would get it. Now, I am managing to read smoother and with less repetition. I always ignored cognitive difficulties because I was so scared of what could happen cognitively. I worked my ass off at getting physically better and I accomplished that, but now I have more work on my brain and it's thinking differently about life, ability, and progression inline. To move forward, slowly and not overly cautiously. Maybe I have been in remission for a while now, but I still think in many ways of what could happen. I guess that never leaves you. Not until we are all cured will that not cross everyone's mind with MS. It is a constant. I am doing well, but what if there is a day when I am not? What if my meds stopped working? That wouldn't happen. I have been on these drugs for sixteen years and starting the double dose is what put me here. Now, an auto-injector, which changed my life so much.

6/28/08

I feel powerful and impactful. I love to make people see another perspective. MS has made me who I am and I am gonna share it with the world – anyone who wants to listen. I like it when people learn something new about life. I like it when people hear me and begin to see the other realities for people. I really like it when people listen and see their own lives differently. It is about the blessings, not the losses.

As I stare at the mountains, I am a little sad that I can't hike them, but very blessed to see them and to be in their presence. Focus on the positive and not the negative. I have so much.

9/20/08

M has been living with me for the last two weeks. She is totally nine months pregnant and overdue. I am getting so stressed that my MS is flaring up. My tremor is worse. My eyes were jumping earlier and I had dizziness. Blah. I had a conversation with my mom and she rocks! She brought me back and told me to take a Xanax and I did. So now I am doing much better. I have been so anxious and impatiently waiting. It is messing with me bad.

Journal Entries: 2009

3/13/09

I am in Telluride and have been here for three days. I took an adaptive ski lesson the day after I arrived. It was amazing. I thought my left leg wouldn't handle it, but it totally did. It felt amazing. It was everything I had hoped for and then some. It was awesome. I felt so strong. I felt like all of the work I have been doing with Jason for the last four years finally paid off in action. It was incredible. The next day I went again, and James came with me. It is so fucking amazing. It is awesome! I am fucking determined to do this and do it well, despite my disability. It felt awesome and I felt like I should be feeling. I loved every second of it. I am feeling so incredible! I have not felt this good in about eleven years. It is truly incredible. Tonight I got to go out to dinner with James and it was incredible. That man blows me away with his drive and determination. He inspires me to get out and do shit. Fuck the MS, I CAN DO IT! After dinner he showed me pictures of him ice climbing with other disabled people. It was incredibly inspiring. I need to bike. James is going to send me a link to good bikes because when I met him this summer, he had the most badass three-wheel bike. I want one. I am blown away by my body and how amazing it is doing. From how I started so many years ago and where I am now is mind-blowing. Jah Bless! It is because of all this hard work I have done and will keep doing. The positive attitude that I have about it all. I am so fucking blessed and so thankful.

Life works in mysterious ways and it is truly incredible to have met James on the streets of Telluride this summer and get to see and spend time with him. My instructor tomorrow is named Hawk Eye. It was funny. But we really are connected on this whole disability thing. The stars aligned for us to meet each other and learn from one another. He gives me strength and I give him hope. Fuck, I caught a fork with my left hand tonight. I am crying now, making the realization that I have gotten so much better. It is fucking awesome. At the same time I realize that James will never get better, but he can. I am so lucky to have this perspective in life already. I cannot believe that I can do these things again. That I caught a fork with my

left hand...holy shit! There is hope. Shit still happens and I not cured, but I am incredible. I have to meet Montel! He inspires me. Now I inspire others. Josh from the support group saw a picture of James and me on top of the mountain and messaged me how big of an inspiration I am to him. I try to be like that with everyone I meet. I am really starting to see my true inner beauty, I think for the first time ever in my life. Shit, at summer camp I got all three awards for being the person who, in a sense, was the coolest. I guess people like me and I am starting to see why. I am a pretty amazing woman. I have not felt this good about myself ever. Life is good.
It is more the good.

8/7/09

On my way to Cali. Life is such a blessing. I really am a lucky woman. I am so stoked to meet Ely and see the family. I brought SkipBo, of course. I land at like 4:15. An hour and forty minutes and I am there. Hatchet is amazing, especially in the airport. He really works with the vest on and as soon as it is off, he is a crazy dog. He is a rock. Just talked to the flight attendant for a while about MS and disability. I love it. This is why it is me. I feel so lucky and blessed. To have Hatchet, my perspective, an awesome sex drive, awesome friends, and a great family. I truly am beyond blessed.

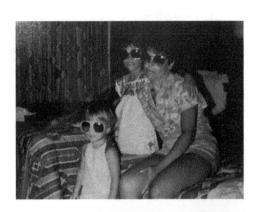

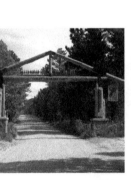

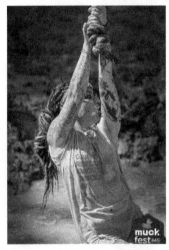

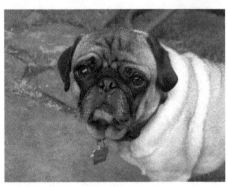

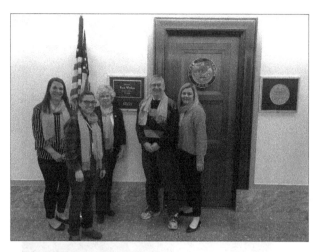

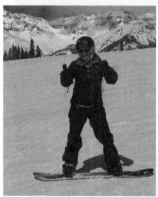

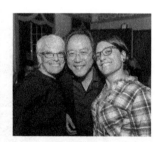

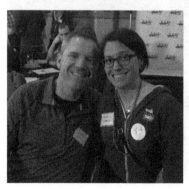

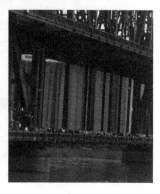

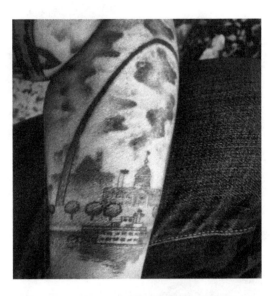

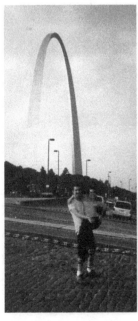

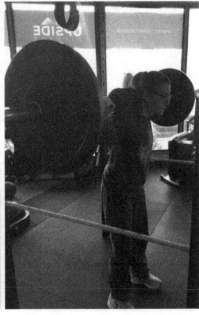

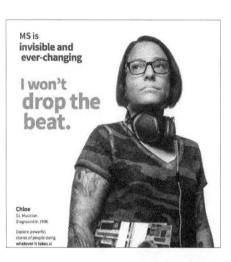

MS is
invisible and
ever-changing

I won't
drop the
beat.

Chloe
D.J. Musician.
Diagnosed in 1998.

Explore powerful
stories of people doing
whatever it takes at.

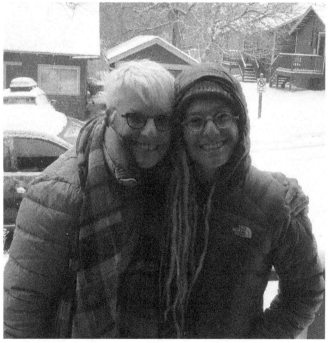

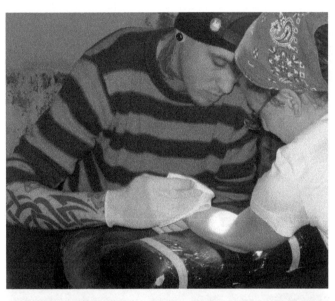

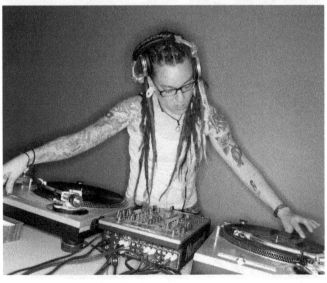

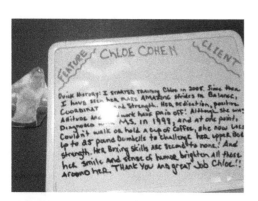

FEATURE CHLOE COHEN CLIENT

QUICK HISTORY! I STARTED TRAINING Chloe in 2005. Since then
I have seen her make AMAZING strides in Balance,
COORDINAT.... ...nd Strength. Her dedication, positive
Attitude and ...work have paid off! Although she was
Diagnosed with M.S. in 1999, and at one point,
Couldn't walk or hold a cup of coffee, she now lifts
up to 25 pound Dumbells to challenge her upper body
strength. Her Boxing skills are second to none! And
her smile and sense of humor brighten all those
around her.. Thank you and great Job Chloe..!!

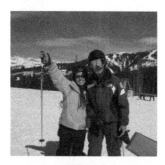

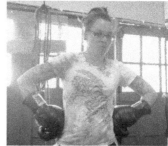

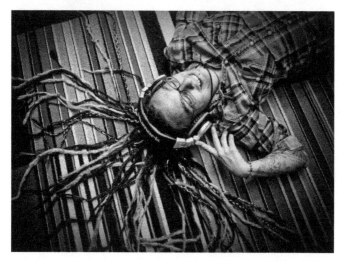

CHAPTER 5

MUSIC

Throughout my life music has been a key for survival. Music came easy to me. I wasn't a prodigy or anything. Yet, the feeling of playing made me complete. How was I going to move forward now with my passion for music? In those beginning years, I had a very hard time listening to people play music from their souls. It always hurt. "That should have been me."

To not have my cello was the biggest devastation to my soul. The cello and the piano were my release of emotion. I could sit at the piano and create a sound that was all my own. The power it held was unmeasurable. The feelings that flowed through me were represented through sound. Through the cello I was able to play pieces of music and express my emotion, my inner person.

In the summer of 2000 I moved to Portland. This is when I would bring back the "turntable love." I bought my second Technic 1200 and I made the mixer my new instrument.

Still playing a lot of hip-hop and a little house, I continued and adapted my style to fit my needs. I had to hold my arm behind my back while the music was playing to make sure it didn't hit the needle. At first I could only go for about fifteen minutes of standing before I had to sit down, but through internet video chat I could have an audience without leaving my home. I began to spin online for people and enjoyed them getting down to my music. I kept at it and continued to improve my skills.

My skills were getting better and I loved finding new records to play. Record shopping was a weekly activity. As time progressed, I started honing my skills even more. I physically got better and worked very hard at carving new pathways in my brain. Having good meds that worked and great doctors, in addition to acupuncture and working out, I began to regain some of what I had lost.

All this contributed to my newer physical and psychological self.

I could spin now for thirty minutes without having to sit down. Soon it was forty-five minutes and recently I have been going over two hours. Time is the biggest healer.

In 2005, I met another DJ who mostly spun house music. I greatly liked his style and it brought me back to my house music roots. Concurrently, I went digital on my turntables by using Serato Scratch Live, but still spinning records. Now I really began to broaden my musical experience. All I had to do was download it. I still use Technic 1200 turntables with vinyl, time coded mats. I did not want to lose that primary skill. This technology that I discovered is now the new way to DJ.

Now, I do play a lot of house, but mostly enjoy mixing it all up from house, hip-hop, 80s, disco, funk, reggae, dancehall, dubstep, and random...I guess they call the electronic with many sub genres "EDM" these days.

I talked with one DJ on a daily basis for a few years. His screen name was Boogieman. I called him Mr. DJ, but his real name was Mike. Mike was from Illinois and eventually came to visit me in Portland. We had an excellent time going record shopping and playing music together. When we cooked together with a longtime friend, I went to grab some condiments off the counter. Something slipped out of my hands and I miraculously caught it with my left hand. My friend's jaw dropped open. I had not done anything like that in eight years. That was the power of the oxytocin. My friend told Mike, "You need to come here every weekend." I smiled in shock from what I had just experienced and how the incredible sex with Mike was making my symptoms lessen and how amazing I felt. For the first time since my diagnosis, I felt confident in my body. I realized that my own self-reflection was making life more difficult. I saw my tremor in a way I had never seen it before. This experience gave me a whole new outlook on the way I viewed my physical limitations and the strength that I had to deal with all of it. This experience would be something that I held onto to remind myself of what is possible and how the way I view myself reflects on the outside.

Mike and I had such a great time together that I had to go back to St. Louis so I could see him again. He only lived a few hours outside of St. Louis and drove on over to hang out. Again, we had an amazing time together. He was the one who greatly changed my view of my tremor.

At the hotel I was staying at, I had a cup of coffee and a hotel room key card. I set my coffee down to use my "good" hand to open the door. He said, "Pick that up and try with your left." I sighed and tried. I couldn't get it. "Keep trying," he said. Frustrated, I kept trying and eventually the door opened. He said, "I knew you could do it." Wow, someone who wasn't going to let me get away from not trying. This was the first positive I experienced of pushing harder.

Mike gave lust a new definition. He turned me on more than any man had ever done. Any extreme emotion is shown through my left arm and my tremor. When I was shaking really badly, he said, "You know, that is hot! I can really tell how excited and into me you are." That was the first time ever where this tremor was a positive thing. The incredible lovemaking that I shared with this man made my symptoms go away for four days. The oxytocin that was released was so powerful. I realized that my own self-reflection was making life more difficult. This experience had given me a whole new outlook on the way I viewed my physical limitations and the strength that I had to deal with all of it. This experience would be something that I held onto to remind myself of what is possible.

In 2008, while at the Northwest World Reggae Festival out in the forest, I really discovered a great tool for me. I needed my coffee and had to stand in a long line for a while. Generally, I would have to sit after standing for more than thirty minutes. The reggae music was bumping loudly throughout the land and I had to move to it. This motion of moving, my reggae sway, if you will, gave me a sense of security on my feet. After about fifteen minutes in line, I realized that if I just kept moving, I could stand for longer. I brought Hatchet with me, which made it easier too. It was an incredible feeling to be outside with nature all around me, the magnificent music pumping through the air.

Laying in the grass on Hatchet, with his vest on, a hippie girl approached me asking about my dog and I told her I had MS. She then said, "Looks like you are in pain, have one of my brownies." I am happy to say that I have never had to deal with any pain with my MS, just other chronic nuances like a constantly shaking left arm and vision issues. I thanked her for the brownie and continued watching the incredible reggae show.

In 2016 I got to meet Yo-Yo Ma in Santa Barbara, California, where my parents live, playing and lecturing at UCSB. It was one of the most amazing experiences of my life. I remember seeing him on *Sesame Street* as a child. Once I picked up the cello in fourth grade, he became an idol of mine. Getting to see him live, the tears just came down. Even as I write this, thinking of how powerful it was, tears are falling. It is all about that emotion, that feeling of creating sound that when he plays, I feel it. I saw how Yo-Yo played his cello through his soul. His face always showed me that he was playing not just with his body, but with his heart and soul. Any musician whose face gets all screwed up when they play is feeling that music in their whole body. Whenever I watched him play, I knew the feeling – that feeling that musicians get when their whole spirit is flowing through them into the instrument. The second time I got to see Yo-Yo perform was again in Santa Barbara, but this time I actually got to meet him. He had met my mother once before where she told him about me and how he needed to tell me to pick up my cello again. I was dumbfounded when I walked into the room and saw him walking around chatting with people. My mother knew the people in charge and asked them if I could meet him. I could.

Holy shit, I was about to meet one of my biggest idols in the world. Someone introduced us and he said hello and hugged me. As he hugged me, he told me to do whatever I want to do. "You don't have to listen to your mother all the time." Did that really happen? After I had that moment, I felt like I got to a new level of peace with the loss of my cello. It really wasn't important that I couldn't play it, but that I could feel it. I did feel it.

Journal Entries: 2010

6/12/10

I know what I have been through and how all of that stuff made me grow into who I am right now. I am lost at the moment and feel very uncertain about the future in different ways than before. The MS gave me a lot of uncertainty, but now this uncertainty is more of just searching for something that fits. My head keeps going and going about this bullshit I am doing to myself. If I want a change, I have to make it happen. I am unsure what I want to be doing or how to do it. I stick to what is comfortable. It is easy to be home, where I can be online and smoke my cannabis. It is so hard to hear all the shitty experiences that happen with people with MS. It is mind-blowing how someone like me and someone who can't walk or who has intense chronic pain have the same disease. It blows me away that all of us who have the same disease are so different with our symptoms and intensity of them. Each person's MS is unique to them. I have yet to meet two people whose MS plays out in the same way.

Journal Entries: 2011

4/11/11

Yesterday was the MSWalk and it was good. K, J, and R came with me. I made it all the way to the Burnside bridge. Mom rocks! I was feeling bad because I only made it that far and was upset. Mom, so beautiful, reminded me of how critical I am of myself and to think about where I was once. That I could now walk that far is huge! It was a very nice wake up call. I then took a nap for an hour.

6/1/11

Today I had another EMDR session. It is intense stuff. We worked specifically on my tremor. It was super intense. I never really realized how many emotions were wrapped up in this MS thing. The tremor does not allow me to hide any emotion. Thank you, Mr. DJ, for giving me a positive with the tremor. You really helped me regain my self-confidence. Where is that person who will do the same for me again?

6/17/11

More EMDR work today that was, again, quite intense. Today we went to the car accident. Lots of pain knowing my body is not my own anymore. I can't control it. I am coming to terms with my brain, mind, and body. Coming to peace with my tremor and the questioning of uncertainty with MS and life. Understanding and believing that my brain and my mind are separate things. Guess I never realized that before. So no matter how fucked my brain is, my mind is still here working 100%. That shit is intense.

6/23/11

EMDR today and it was pretty intense as always. Learning to let it go, be at peace with my brain and learn a new way. Playing new tapes in my head that I am a safe driver and can do it. Fear is starting to subside a bit.

7/21/11

...This EMDR is some powerful stuff. Today we went to the car accident and the wall that I hit. She said something that was so powerful. That wall saved my life. I had never been able to think of that wall in any other way than a

death trap, but holy shit, it really did save my life. I am feeling safer and more comfortable when driving. P is so sweet and hugs me. It is so amazing what she has done for me and how amazing I feel about myself. But I am looking for something more...

CHAPTER 6

EXERCISE AND ACUPUNCTURE

*I*n 2007, I started working out and quickly got a trainer to help guide me through. I had never worked out in a gym before. At first, they hooked me up with this jock guy who was ready to get me in shape. He talked about football and strippers and I felt he didn't really understand what I needed, being that I had not used my left arm in almost ten years and he clearly had no understanding of what MS was. I worked out with him for maybe six months and then he moved to another gym and handed me off to another trainer. This new trainer understood my limitations and was ready to take on the challenge.

Jason Thomas, my new trainer, had no real prior knowledge of MS until he met me. I showed up and it presented him with something new, challenging, and different and he was ready to take it on. Because I had held my arm behind my back for so long, he knew this was the first challenge.

He began by reminding me to bring my arm forward. It was so natural for me to hold it behind my back because I was self-conscious and scared that it could hit something or knock it over. When it was behind my back, I could ignore it better, not having the visual or the constant shaking, but after time I became more aware of bringing my arm in front of me. I was really trying hard to learn how to adapt back into using my left arm.

This working out presented quite the challenge on so many levels. The fatigue I would feel after a one hour session had me knocked out for the rest of the day. My mind was awake, but my body was not working with my mind. The fatigue was a major symptom that could not be ignored and was constantly present. Luckily for me, Jason was a very smart man with his understanding of the human body. He had been an athlete in high school and then studied health and fitness in college and really knew what he was doing. He had the knowledge to get me started on this new journey. After about a year of consistent workouts I slowly was getting less fatigued and was definitely not hiding my arm behind my back as much. Jason really became someone close and a brother-type in my life. Jason understood my body and how it worked with the neurological condition of MS. He constantly challenged my brain along with my muscles. He understood that this was my brain, and not my muscles, fighting. It started with a simple movement of acting like I was picking up my pug and placing him on a shelf on the other side of my body. Because I had not really used my left arm much at all, this movement was reminding my brain that my arm was still there and does work. Those initial workouts were so brutal. I was crushed after every workout and couldn't quite understand how this was helping me when it made me feel so fatigued after. This was so not easy and I wanted to stop, but I knew that with time it might get easier.

It took about a year before I stopped getting so fatigued after and actually started noticing that my energy was improving. I worked on balance and coordination with exercises that constantly challenged me. Jason was constantly switching things up with different activities and exercises to challenge my brain. I call this "brain sweat," when my brain is sweating hard and gets mushy and I have to really fully concentrate on what I am doing. This is how I have created new pathways in my brain. We have done so many exercises that challenge my brain way more than my body. He always asked me questions, about music, mostly, while I was trying to complete tasks that made my brain work super hard. He had little round disks that each had letters or numbers on them. He would yell out an animal and tell me to jump to the letter it started with. "Chicken," jump to C, "Elephant," jump to E. This was making me use my brain in many ways at the same time. Neuroplasticity is a very real thing and I am a prime example of that.

When I started with him, I couldn't jump onto a short platform without falling. My left side was constantly the challenge, learning again how to use it and trust it. Learning to trust my body was very challenging. All the fears of falling for so many years made this fear very real. Many times I said, there is no way my body will let me do this. Generally, I failed on my first attempt, but I always got it down by the end. Being the soccer player that I was, I was competitive with myself. I had to finish each exercise right. If I didn't get it right the first five times, I would do it as many more times as I needed to until I got it right, even though Jason told me to stop. Anything that involved balance and coordination made me nervous.

During a workout Jason would pull out a simple step stool and put a foam square below it. I was to stand on the foam and take two steps up onto the step stood. One foot and the other. Then back down. One, two. Down to the foam.

A simple motion, but it challenged my brain and was actually carving new pathways in my brain. I have always been the hardest on myself through this whole battle, but I also know that without all that determination I would not be anywhere near where I am now. I will forever keep pushing myself, not too hard but hard enough to see change. From where I was once to where I am now, I am truly blown away. I wish others could experience all the amazement that I have all the time in living with MS. I feel so grateful for everything in my life. Not only was I gaining strength back in my arm, but Jason was challenging my nervous system and working on carving new connections in my brain.

I have worked with him consistently for so many years and regained so much function that I really know if there is a will there is a way and that finding the right person to help guide you is essential. Jason is a brilliant personal trainer who always makes it fun. I love playing soccer. I was not an amazing player, but I was good and had so much fun playing. I had always played left fullback and my left side was my strong side – in fact, I played cello using my left arm. Knowing that I was a soccer player from age six through high school, he fed my athletic drive.

Jason understood my energy and heat issues, so he always made sure I drank water and didn't overheat. I stayed cool, hydrated, and eventually was actually gaining energy from my workouts. It really became the biggest, most positive life change I had made so far.

After a few years of battling in the gym, I started really seeing the rewards. I wasn't as exhausted after a workout. More often I had energy to complete my day. I began to do some heavy lifting in the gym with heavy weights. Maybe Jason just wanted me to become aware of how truly strong I am or just was curious about how much I could lift, but I went from lifting eighty pounds to 130 pounds. Now, I do two weeks heavy lifting followed by two weeks off with regular circuit training.

I started boxing with Jason maybe five years ago and I love it. Just a little punching and kicking made me feel like a badass. It was cardio work, which I really didn't like, but because it was all action, I didn't even realize how fast my heart rate was. It also makes me feel like I am one strong, powerful woman. I am a small woman, barely five feet tall, and this was making me feel giant. I know that if I had to, I could seriously hurt someone with my wicked uppercut. I don't think I would ever really hurt someone, but it feels good knowing that I could and that I can defend myself if I need to. I have gained so much self-confidence from all this work. I really have proven to myself that I can do anything that I put my mind to. I can actually physically see my strength and power. None of this work has been easy at all, but the rewards far outweigh the difficulties I had initially. Every week I have at least two powerful moments at the gym where I reflect back on how impossible this would have been to do even six years ago. Those are amazing moments. I have had a few moments of tears of joy being in shock about what I have just done. I am strong. I am powerful. I am a beast.

Jason changed my life. It was really hard to make the progress I have, but with the help of Jason, I have done it. He gave me confidence and strength in dealing with my MS. I am my toughest critic and constantly want to challenge myself more just to see how far I can go. I regained the use of my arm. The feeling of holding a glass with my left hand now and not having it shake all the liquid out is mind-blowing. Going from not being able to wash my face with two hands, not being able to tie shoes or cut my food to being where I am at now is incredible. I can do all those things now. I can do more now than I could ever do before, even before the MS. Again, you don't know what you have until you lose it. Well, I lost it and now it is back. I wish more people could understand what that feels like.

Not only is Jason an exceptional personal trainer, he is also a great father, husband, and fisherman. He is definitely the brother I never had and there is constant humor throughout our workouts. Too many times I have had to stop mid-movement to bend over and laugh. There is always conversation about nineties music or movies. He showed up to my fortieth birthday as a cowboy and I totally did not recognize him and thought, "Who invited that guy?" It was Jason dressed as Cowboy Carl, ready to join in the fun with my friends and family. There are always lots of laughs and fun times while working out and when we get to socialize. The private jokes constantly thrown out at the right time will always make me laugh.

Over the years of working out with Jason, I regained so much of what I had lost and my attitude has greatly shifted. I will forever keep pushing and trying to do things that I am scared of and that I doubt I could do. When I do them and prove myself wrong, the feeling of amazement is unmeasurable. I am strong and capable. After so many years of self-doubt and fear, I have learned that I can do almost anything. I have confidence that I lost for a good fifteen years. Every little step I took got me closer to taking the leaps and bounds that I am taking now.

In July of 2013, I did the MuckFest for MS with my wonderful friend Lucas Gamlin. It is an obstacle course through mud in St. Louis. I told myself it would prove to me how strong I was now after ten years of disability and challenging myself physically every week with my trainer for the last eight years. I looked forward to seeing what my body could do. After eight years of pushing my body in ways I never thought I would or could, I could now be an able-bodied person in the world and keep pushing more for all those people who can't push anymore. I did it. MuckFest, all 5K. All the obstacles seemed easy. I felt overly prepared. And I think I was. It showed me how strong I was/had become. It blew me away. There was a long time there where I never thought this could happen. It's amazing how coordinated I had become.

Around the same time I started to work out, I also started acupuncture. I had done it once back in 2003 and my tremor stopped while the needles were in. It freaked me out so much that I never went back, but after many years I finally did. This new woman, Rayna Jacobson, was a healer and I felt it. Not only did she do acupuncture, but she also did Reiki and energy work. She had been a nurse for many years before she studied at the College of Oriental Medicine and really honed her healing skills. She was a self-proclaimed Jew-Bu, Jewish Buddhist, which connected with my background as a Reform Jew who wasn't really a religious person, but definitely a spiritual one. She was a healer with a special touch of spirituality which really brought us together closer.

When I started with Rayna, as I was lying on the table I could feel my arm bouncing around, but once the needles were in it calmed. I had not felt this calm in many years, and it was so amazing to feel. During the time the needles were in, there was a peace to my body that I had never felt since my diagnosis. This was incredible and I knew that it was going to be something that I had needed for a long time but had denied its power. I was going for acupuncture every two weeks, mostly to help with my fatigue, as well as my tremor. Rayna understood my limitations and was dedicated to helping relieve me from as much as she could through her practices. Eventually, I could go three weeks without it, but I always felt the fatigue creeping in toward the end of the third week. After staying consistent with my treatments, I started to really notice the fatigue being lifted off of me. I felt amazing after every appointment and knew this would now become a lifelong experience that I had to have. I was so grateful to discover acupuncture because I could now live a more fulfilling life without so much fatigue.

I worked with Rayna until 2017, when she retired and I found another acupuncturist. I know no one will be as wonderful as she was, but those needles were keeping me functioning in a way that I once thought was impossible.

It is the walls of fear that I have had to break down and continue to break down. The tapes I keep playing in my head have now changed. I can now actually see my strength and power. For all the years of self-doubt and fear I have reached a point in my life where know I can get through any obstacle put before me. I have regained so much and keep on pushing myself to see how far I can go.

To finally get relief from severe fatigue and get a sense of calmness throughout my body through my exercise and my acupuncture is something that I know took many years to build. I know that these things will forever be in my life because it is essential to continue on this path I am on. The future is bright. Brighter than it has ever been in twenty years.

Journal Entries: 2012

3/14/12

Fear from what I once experienced seems to be the main thing that I feel when trying something again that I once couldn't do, even though I know how strong and capable I am now. At my parents' house there is a pool with a fourteen-inch concrete ledge around it. I have always feared walking around the pool on the ledge. Watching other people walk around it with no problem. Watching my friend do a handstand on the edge, I thought I would always be watching others have no problem with it. This fear is what was holding me back from making those steps. What if I fell off the edge? What if my body wouldn't do what I was telling it to do? After ten years of uncertainty about how my body would react to situations that were not safe, I finally walked the edge. Just one step at a time. I keep testing myself to prove to myself that I can do these things. So I took five steps and took a deep breath, telling myself I could do it. I took five more steps, on the edge. I made it to the end of one side. Proud of myself and a little emotional, I told myself I could make it all the way down. One foot in front of the other. I see how much my brain is working with my body. The second I have a thought that I could fall, my balance is off. I can catch myself right away and continue to challenge myself. Then, I make it to the other end of the other side, stare at what I just did with relief, with confidence and happiness. I look at this experience as part of this whole healing process.

7/7/2012

Talked to Mike T. today for the first time in like six or seven years. He was one of the first males in our support group when we started it years ago. He had PPMS (Primary Progressive MS), which there are no meds for and which is really is the most debilitating kind of MS. We, the support group, which consisted of a max of five or six people, watched him quickly lose more and more function. When he started coming to the group, he had optic neuritis and used a cane. We bonded over what it was like when the earth just moved from under your feet, randomly. He was probably the first person in my life who related to me on that level besides Laura, who could relate as well. Very quickly he went from a guy who used a cane to using a wheelchair and becoming less and less independent. The last time I saw him here in Portland, six years ago, he was bedridden and hopeless. Every time I think of him, I get so emotional. This is what makes life with MS the hardest. Watching people struggle and decline with their physical mobility, function, and hope. This is why I always fight for MS and why I write and why voices need to be heard. I may be only one voice, but my voice has already been spread to many. The reason why I have made MS my mission in life in so many ways is because I am someone who knows the other side, who knows the struggle, who cares. It will always be my lifelong cause to educate and enlighten people with the wisdom that MS taught me. Only through all that struggle and challenge did I find my strength, courage, and hope. The MS has carved a path in my life that has led me to where I am now. Because of Mike and so many others I have met since him, I can't stop the fight until there is a cure for all forms of MS. It will happen. Maybe by the time this book gets published, there will be a cure for MS. That might be a little hopeful, because I hope to have this book out faster than science moves, but I know that it is in the near future with how far they have come since I was diagnosed.

10/12/12

Crazy to look back and be shocked by where I am now. To go from being disabled and in constant question of the future to now not worrying about what physically might happen. I am free from the burden of the constant questioning of what my future might hold. Not having the center of my life be MS and only worrying about regular worries in life. Will I find a relationship in the future? For so many years I was not looking for any serious relationships because of my fear of the future and not trusting my body. Now, I think I am ready to meet someone special, but I have no idea how to get out. I am so comfortable in my home, on the computer, with my animals, that I have not pushed myself out too much. I guess it's time for me to do that, but I am slow on the uptake and find it easier to just stay put, even though I know there is nothing holding me back other than myself. I guess I am just scared. I don't know what of. Probably has more to do with being alone.

Hard to get myself to do things alone. I don't have much motivation to get out when alone.

10/14/12

Will I have children? Will I adopt children? Do I want to put my body through the stress of pregnancy? Do I want to experience that? After my diagnosis, I was so depressed about being a woman and not going to have a child. It scared me. I like walking. I like seeing clearly. Would I want to risk all that for a child of my own when there are so many children that need homes? I know ultimately I would like to have a partner who shares the responsibility. Guess I will cross that bridge when I come to it. Would it be worth the risks to have my own genetics in my child? Could I pass on the MS? I can't imagine having a child with...wait. I would be able to deal with anything that my child might experience. No matter if they were mine genetically or not. There are so many issues in this world. All the child needs is love. I think I am more on the adoption kick, but anything is possible.

Journal Entries: 2013

1/20/13

I started using the Avonex pen last week. Holy shit it is easy! I have been needing this for so many years. It is awesome. So I will go to the clinic on Monday for one last shot to use the last injection they have there. So now that the clinic won't be a part of my routine anymore, I need to find something to fill that space.

4/18/13

As I train for the MuckFest, I notice how fear is my biggest obstacle. I get so fearful when I want to try new and challenging things. After ten years of being careful and not pushing too hard, I find it is more a mental thing than a physical thing. After years of falling, or having the earth fall out from under me, I have learned to be more careful with my steps and my physical body. Now that my coordination and my strength have improved so much, the harder part is working on my mind, that I can do things. I have to change the fears of falling, stumbling or hurting myself into I

CAN DO IT! Moving from the fears of all the what-ifs and all the questioning, I am blown away almost every day by how different my life is now that I have changed so much physically. This mental challenge is just as difficult, it seems.

11/21/13

In a session with Debera, it started with me holding my hands out while listening to monks chanting and water flowing. My left arm represented how the old me felt and the right was the person I feel I am now. I slowly brought them together at my own slow pace. When my hands clasped together it was way powerful. Like the new me is always there or would be there for the old me and the new me. Can't really describe the feeling, but it was almost like a click when my hands touched. She also talked about the gate in my heart. How I need to keep it closed until I absolutely am ready to open it. Not really sure right now Then tonight I drove myself to the support group for the first time in years. I did it. There were only a couple moments of fear, but I did it. I am feeling the best I have felt in years.

12/18/13

Harsh losses quickly create a different path. The path was constantly moving in different directions, all around, up and down, back and forth, left and right, sometimes in and out. The focus wasn't on the losses or the grief, but on powering on forward and being strong. I put that grief, that sadness in my back pocket. It is time to take it out and look at it again. The pain of living with a chronic illness, of knowing your brain and your body are forever fucked. There is no repair.... WAIT! Now I have made it easy. This is crazy. All those questions and uncertainties have changed. Time heals, time takes forever, time moves too fast. In the moment, it is all the same amount of time. As I wait to see what the future holds, I no longer have to deal with all the uncertainties of MS anymore. I don't even know. I tried to be creative, just flow. I think it is just bedtime. Trying to live in the moment and in the present.

CHAPTER 7

INK

My tattoos tell stories of my life. The first tattoo I got was during my first few months away at college. At eighteen, my roommate and I went and got them together. I drew mine up of a Celtic knot with a star in the center over my womb. It was to bless my children. It being my first tattoo, I really didn't realize how painful it was until many years later when I went to touch it up again. A couple years later I went and got a couple of Stars of David on my calves to represent my family and heritage. I waited another couple years and got a lotus with an infinity symbol in the center of the back of my neck. The infinity symbol was made out of two bass clefs to represent my cello and the fact that music is infinite in my soul. I can forever and always hear it and feel it. I felt so amazing after that tattoo, like I was on top of the world. I think it was the location, because I never felt that way after a tattoo again. The itch for a new tat starts pretty much as soon as you are healed from the last one.

I was getting needles for my own pleasure rather than the intermuscular injections, which I never wanted. I wanted to take some of the power away from needles, and getting tattooed gave me a bit more of a sense of control over the needles. I chose these needles, rather than feeling like I did not have a choice about my injections. My mother always said I had a choice, but really, being as physically messed up as I was, I knew medicine was a good thing, as much as it sucked. Getting a little more ink always made me feel good. The dopamine and endorphins released with pain is a powerful high and I think that is what I really craved.

I managed to wait another year, but it was time. I went and got the kanji symbol for harmony on my right arm. Harmony was crucial in my life. When I hear a smooth harmony it brings chills to my body and sometime tears to my eyes. I couldn't see the artwork on my neck and knew how beautiful it was, so I went back to the same artist to put some flowers around the kanji symbol. I could see his artwork all the time now. On the last round of color on the flowers, the artist said to me, "You are going to have a sleeve before you know it." I said, "Oh, no way. That won't happen." It didn't take too long for the itch to start again, saying, "You *need* more ink."

I loved scuba diving, the ocean, and sea life. I decided I wanted saltwater fish on my forearm. I knew the skill this man had, so I told him what I wanted and he drew it out and we started again on finishing my right sleeve. After a few sessions, it was done. The inside of my right arm was still blank, and I was waiting because I thought it was going to be so painful. I had set up another few appointments to complete the right arm. My appointment was shortly after my car accident and I was still very discombobulated from the experience. I don't remember the physical pain because I was still a mess from the accident. These new flowers represented my dogs who I had lost in the accident. Whenever I looked at them, I would kiss my arm, telling my dogs I missed them.

Because of my tremor, I could not get my left arm tattooed until I went to Holland for the first time. My friend and I were going to get matching tattoos. I really wanted my new tattoo on my left arm, and I told the guy what I wanted. I told him I wanted it on my left arm, but that I shake pretty bad. He said, "No problem. We will hire two fat men to sit on your arm if we have to." I love the Dutch. He then went back and talked to the tattooer. He wanted to take it on. This guy was also disabled – he had spina bifida

– so I think he understood why I wanted it on my left arm and what it meant to me to have it there. Not only was this guy disabled too, but so, so good looking. I don't remember any pain because I was looking at him the whole time. They also let me smoke a joint before I sat in the chair to calm my tremor before we started. The Dutch understood the medicinal properties of cannabis. With this symbol I put the word "irie," which means positivity, to remind me to always look at the positives in life. Reggae music always helped me find positive feelings when I was down. Life really is all about the irie vibes and staying in a positive mindset. Bob Marley's lyrics have always given me a bright, warm glow over my life. Bob was someone who reminded people of the power of love and how we are all connected. The lyrics of "Three Little Birds," "Positive Vibration," and "The Sun is Shining" really were mantras that rang through my head to remind myself of all that I have and want to be in the future.

The following year I got a scorpion on my back to represent the Scorpio that I am. But, because I was going through a spell of fatigue, I was taking medication to keep me more awake and what that did was electrify my nervous system, so about ten minutes into the tattoo I had to stop. I had never had a tattoo be so painful. I told the artist that I had to stop, but that as soon as I was off this medication I would be back to finish. After a couple weeks I went back and finished the outline. I returned later for the color and it turned out to be one beautiful tattoo. For me it is all about the artist and spreading my tattoo love all around. There was an incredible artist from whom I wanted to get a St. Louis waterfront image. He was very excited to not be doing a Portland scene and was looking forward to creating this image on my left arm. My tremor had calmed a bit compared to what it was like before. This tattoo represented all the love for my hometown and all the special relationships I have to people and places there.

I then got a hummingbird on the top of my left arm. I love hummingbirds and they remind me of my grandmother. As much as she didn't understand tattoos, I think at this point she finally got to see the artistry of tattoos because she loved hummingbirds so much. I only had one and my friend said to me, "You need two more so you can have three little birds for Bob." He was right. I needed two more birds to complete this section of my arm. I later followed it up with more flowers around the birds. These flowers attract hummingbirds and really completed that section of tattoos.

I had to get ink to represent my Dutch love, so I went to another artist and had him do a windmill with tulips on my lower left arm, next to my irie tattoo. I had him add some clouds around the St. Louis Arch and fill up some of the empty space.

Soon enough I finally got my MS tattoo. This tattoo was a butterfly made out of the MS ribbon, colored with red, green, and yellow, again to represent the power of positivity. I had three words in Hebrew around the ink: hope, strength, and courage, because that is what it takes to live with a chronic illness. I wrote those words in Hebrew to represent my heritage and family ties. This was a powerful tattoo that really clarified how I got to this point in my life.

In 2015, one of my best friends passed away from a suicide. This was the most brutal death I have experienced. I had only known her for a couple years, but in that time we got super close and she really became my right hand man. We would go to shows together, play cards, and mostly laugh. We became really close really fast and I was so happy to have a friend who really made me feel so lucky to have a friend like her. She was not a happy woman. I really had no idea. Clearly, she was really good at putting on her game face. I had no idea how depressed and miserable she truly was. That day she contacted her friends and told them she was done with life. I really was in disbelief at how hard life was for her.

I was devastated, as were most of her friends. Losing her was one of the hardest things I have gone through in my life. This just made me want to fight harder for my own life. I know I will never have a friend like her again and I was tortured by that fact. There was nothing that was going to take away that loss, but I had to represent my love for her, so I got another tattoo in honor of her. I got a big black widow on my back to remember her by, because one time we were camping and she was convinced there was a spider on her and was scared to death of spiders. My friends and I had never laughed so hard at her circling, wiping her back and chest, screaming, trying to get the spider off. There was no spider, she was just paranoid. I felt like having a big spider on my back would always remind me of that night and the camping trip that was so epic for our friendship. She was now with me forever.

The next tattoo was one of Mount Wilson in Colorado. My house in Telluride has always been my favorite place on Earth. From anywhere in the house you have a view of this mountain that has always brought me joy. Mount Wilson was so beautiful from the house and I wanted to have that with me every day. I found another artist who put it on my left wrist. Now, I could see that mountain whenever I wanted.

I still have a lot of open space on my body and know that by the time I am fifty, I will have a lot of my body covered. I have been getting tattooed for over twenty years and can only imagine what will happen in the next twenty. It is an addiction. No pain, no gain.

Journal Entries: 2014

1/19/14

Feel like I am never going to have children or find a life partner. Maybe I am impatient or feeling doubtful. Being with my parents on their forty-fifth anniversary is a beautiful thing. It reminds me how alone I am and have been for so long. I know that things will change eventually, but right now, I feel very alone. I have managed my MS and all the bad stuff I dealt with for ten years, but I never have found what I am really looking for. True love. This is what we all need. I have so much love from my parents and friends, but there is a more special love I am looking for, which has to exist somewhere. I am capable of taking care of children, I think. I do need ten hours sleep every night. Because I can get sleep, I am doing better physically than I would be if I couldn't get the sleep that I need.

3/22/14

I have been in Telluride for four days. I love it here so much. The idea of losing this house kills me, but I don't think it will happen for a while. I went snowboarding yesterday for the first time in six years and it was mind-blowing. I felt like MS almost never happened. It felt so good to get that feeling again. Wow! I thought skiing again was awesome, but getting on that board again and actually carving the snow heel to toe felt amazing It showed me how awesomely this training with Jason plays out on the mountains. Holy shit, I am one strong woman. I really am in shock at how well my body works. That was some powerful shit. My instructor, Dead Head Aaron, was impressed with my balance. My fucking balance! For years it was shit. Wow, it felt incredible. Today I went back out with him and another guy and it was fun. We went up higher. I could not stay on the T-Bar lift. It was totally awkward, so we hiked up. Holy shit! I did that and I did that much better than I thought. It did feel like I was seventeen again.

7/12/14

As I sit in St. Louis ready and pumped for the MuckFest, I must remind myself how strong I really am. The heat is what I worry about, but I have learned a lot over the last sixteen years about how to deal with it. I bought a cooling neck wrap with ice packs in it to keep me cool. We will be jumping in water and mud, so I know that will help greatly. I am tough and will respect my body's wishes.

When I did the MuckFest in St. L., I was so emotional. Probably more than most people there. I look forward to showing people a positive picture of MS. I am sure there will be other MSers there. Going through that finish line for me is gonna be amazing and I keep focusing on that. Today, hiking over all the branches, I kept telling myself this was preparation for the obstacles. We will see what tomorrow brings and it will be good. Life is always so amazing here in Telluride, my home away from home. So many experiences here. So many huge life experiences with MS.

7/24/14

I went to Bluegrass again and it is mind-blowing looking back at past Bluegrass experiences and how much I have changed. I am slowly but properly becoming that person I was to be. That I am. I have gained so much knowledge through this whole experience and I greatly see it as a blessed perspective on life. Knowing what I know and learning so much so young, I look at my future and am excited to see what I can/will do next. I feel like in the last six years I have grown so much physically, as well as mentally. I have confidence and I feel so able and determined to make a change in my life in whatever way I need. Now, I am seeing such positivity in my life and know I will affect many people with my words. I've got to stop putting so much pressure on wording everything right.

9/2014

In Texas for Grammy's ninetieth birthday. Last night a beautiful party with thirteen of the symphony players and 250 people. Amazing family all around. I am so lucky or blessed to have this family and this health. If it wasn't for people like Grammy Roz they wouldn't be as close to a cure. I couldn't have felt more amazing. Walking around, standing, schmoozing with all the people. Three separate times people came up to me about my speech in 2008 for the MS Society. Amazing. For the first time in sixteen years, I could stand for such a long period of time and do what I always wanted to do with all these people. I felt on top of the world. These people heard and felt me. All these people knew my story through Grammy and saw me standing up there without assistance. I felt so lucky to be standing up there giving everyone a different perspective on life. I feel honored to be in the position I am in and nothing feels better then showing everyone how incredible my life is and how far I have come.

9/10/2014

Almost sixteen years later and I am doing stuff most able-bodied people couldn't do. Every time I work out with Jason I set a personal goal to create new pathways. I am constantly challenging myself and seeing how far I can push myself. Almost every time I am doing something challenging, I try and get it right at least once. Even after Jason has said stop, I must get one perfect. It took a good two years or so before I could feel the benefit of working out. I was so exhausted every time and needed a lot of rest afterward. After about two years I could start to get actual energy from my workouts. It has become such a regular thing for me that when I don't do it, I feel like something is missing. Every time I work out, I am in shock at how far I have come. Doing things now I could never have done before. Constantly challenging my brain.

Journal Entries: 2015

1/29/15

Feeling real good after a successful meeting tonight with the biggest group we have had, ever. There were thirty people. It is amazing to see all the strength in everyone and how we all are there for each other. Pretty awesome stuff. This whole MS bull is behind me in so many ways. I am amazed when I step back from myself at how far I have come. Every month I feel so amazed by how I feel when they hear my story. Especially those who have gone through a lot themselves. I thought a lot about Mike T. tonight. Has he pushed through? Just sending the irie vibes out to him tonight.

1/31/15

For the first time in almost sixteen years, I was able to coordinate my left and right side at the same time, jumping on and off a foam square. I couldn't believe it while I was doing it. I began to cry and get emotional. It was so freaking powerful! Jason said, "I've seen tears of fear and of pain, but these tears are joy. It's a first for this gym. Congratulations!" I felt so freaking amazing! Just to look back over the last few years and see how incredibly I am doing. This shit I am doing I once never thought possible. Hiking, snowboarding, skiing, the MuckFest, and even knitting. Wow! I really have done more than I give myself credit for. I am just blown away by the power of the brain. Today I found out that one of the members of our support group died. I still don't know any details, but it is really sad. Why am I doing so well and then there are people like Angel, Sarah, Laura, and Mike who just keep suffering? So it is just crazy.

2/5/15

Crazy to look back and be shocked by where I am now. To go from being disabled and in constant question of my future and now, not worrying about what physically might happen. I am free from the burden of the constant questioning of what my future might hold. Not having the center of my life be MS and only worrying about regular worries in life. Will I find a relationship in the future? For so many years I was not looking for any serious relationships because of my fear of the future. Now, I am ready to meet someone special, but I have no idea how to get out. I am so comfortable in my home, on my computer, with my animals, that I have not pushed out too much. I guess it is time for me to do that, but I am slow on the uptake and find it easier to just stay put, even though I know there is nothing holding me back other than myself. I guess I am just scared. I don't know of what. It probably has more to do with being alone. Hard to get myself to do things alone. I don't have much motivation to get out when alone.

Being single for so many years, I am very comfortable being alone. It kind of scares me to think of sharing my life with someone. I guess I don't put too much out there to change it or too much effort to meet new people. I just sit at home and talk to people online all the time or I am on my turntables in the basement.

Why is it so difficult for me to push myself out there alone? I can do it. I am just scared. Of what? It is just a pattern in my brain that I keep enforcing. I've got to create new tapes, records in my head. Stop with all this old stuff and try and push forward in different ways. I did it with my body and now is the time to do it mentally and step out of my box.

2/8/15

I have begun to train for the MuckFest in St. Louis in July. Feel like I am at bootcamp. It blows me away how far I have come physically. I am so thankful that I pushed myself through all the pain and struggle. I have gained a new life and I am constantly trying to make it better through this hard work. To think when I started to train with Jason eight years ago, I didn't even use my left arm at all. Last week I was doing things I could have never done. Intense three-minute intervals. My brain gets mushy when I start pushing myself that hard. I am constantly forgetting how to do the exercise or which side I am on. Brain sweat is what I call it. I feel like I am carving away new pathways when I do these challenging physical things.

2/18/15

I am finally getting my MS tattoo. I decided on a butterfly made out of the MS ribbon. The colors will be red, green, and yellow for my love of Bob. In Hebrew I will put hope, strength, and courage around it. Finally. Most of my ink represents my struggles, but this is my power MS ink. Not gonna start it until mid-March, but I am ready for that itch to be scratched. Life moves forward, things change, time passes. It is what we make of it. I am taking my baby steps with things, but I am taking steps and I am moving forward positively. I am satisfied.

4/15/15

Being with Ely and Myles (my niece and nephew) is the best thing in the world. They love me so much and tell me and there is nothing better. I love kids. I love being an aunt. I see children in my future at some point. I will adopt children, they will be mine and the love will be ever-present. I am on the adoption kick because I don't want to move backward with my health. However children enter my life, they will be loved. That is all you need. All I need is love and music. Last night siting in front of the symphony, I was so happy to listen and not reflect on myself and my loss of the cello. I couldn't have been more joyful to listen to them play. That will never be lost on me.

Being with my family and seeing all the love was truly incredible. That is all we need — love, family, and our health. I am so bleeesssss- seeeedddd to have all this love around me. I am so lucky.

So much to say about love. I have been quite alone for many years but now, I feel like I am ready to let someone into my heart. My twenties were spent disabled and tired. My family and friends really bring me joy and send me love. I have been single through pretty much all of my MS battle. It would have been nice to have someone, but I didn't and I was too focused on myself. Because all of my self-confidence was lost back in 1998, I spent all this time trying to rebuild what was lost.

6/13/15

Just say what I am feeling. I am feeling lost and questioning my abilities. I can't seem to force myself out of this house. I have been here since Friday. It is Monday and the only interactions I had with people were online, at the dispensary, and when I looked at a bike.

I've got to remind myself of all the strengths I do have and all that I have learned through the last sixteen years. I somehow got through all that needle fear. I've got to see what I have accomplished. That speech I gave in Texas really was mind-blowing. What year was that? 2003? I really rock at public speaking. Why don't I do any of that?

What is my goal right now? Other than getting out of this funk I am in. What do I want to do? I don't know. I should use these communication skills I have somehow. I use them every month at our meetings, but not with anything unrelated to MS. I don't know what else to speak about. I have been rolling through the years, getting stronger and more confident. Somehow I got through college with all the bullshit of MS. Somehow I went skiing and snowboarding. I did those things. I forced myself to start to work out. I walked into Art from the Heart (AFTH). I did it and, so I know if there is a will there is a way, but I can't figure out where I want to go. How do I progress forward? What do I really want to do? I gotta find something that draws me in. Do I go back to school for special education? Do I find writing groups somewhere? How do I find them? I need to do something with people. Talking to people. It isn't about disability anymore. It isn't about sickness anymore. What is it about? Finding peace? What is my mission now? I know how many people I have affected by speaking. I know each one of them heard what I said. What is just that good, but bigger? I guess this book. Writing is a form of communication. Yet there is a little bit more interpreta-

tion on the reader's part. When you speak, the audience hears what is meant through inflection and intonation. Writing gives the reader an opportunity to understand with a smaller amount of personal touch from the speaker.

6/14/15

Volunteering at Art from the Heart has given me a new perspective on disability. Getting to do art and communicate with all these amazing people and share in their lives is astounding. The hearts of these people are so huge. Getting a view of life from someone with Down syndrome or autism really makes me see the overflowing love and care all these people have for people. And it makes me realize how lucky, blessed, thankful, and grateful I really am. Couldn't be here without my amazing parents, super awesome friends, and an awesome personal trainer. I have gone through it. I experienced it. And what now? If I don't have the MS to worry about, what pushes me forward now? How do I force myself out of my comfort zone?

Push forward. Keep climbing higher. Take some risks. Try something new. Write it. Uncertainty. Racking my brain trying to think.

6/23/15

I want to get married but I can't seem to meet any nice straight boys. With no MS ruling my life, what is my mission? I spend too much time thinking about the what-ifs. Live in the present, move from the past, and move forward to the future with the wisdom of what I've learned through all these years. It is time for me to get out of this comfort zone. Learn how to take risks and give myself to the world. No more worrying every day what's going to happen next. I still seem to just sit here waiting for something to happen. I trained myself to stay home and be comfortable. Even after six years of not having to worry about anything happening with my MS, I still hold myself back and don't push as hard as I could to meet that man of my dreams. Patience. I'm tired of waiting but know it will be well worth the wait and whoever it is will love me regardless of the MS or any other ailment.

11/21/15

It is time to treat myself to a break in the world. I've got to stop beating myself down so much. I've got to gain more dedication to getting out in the world. Moving forward through life. I just turned thirty-seven and I'm confused by how fast I got here. I always thought by the time I was thirty-five I would be married, have a career, and children of my own. I am happy where I am in life, but I still feel something is missing, something I don't know yet.

CHAPTER 8

NEXT STEPS

*I*n April 2017, I started a new medication that was now a twice a year infusion. No more needles! No more side effects. It has totally changed my life. For the first time in twenty years I felt like totally different person. It didn't make me feel bad. The first half dose I had went pretty smoothly. It was a six-hour process. They give you Benadryl and steroids to start you off to avoid any allergic reactions, but my throat got itchy anyway and I started having an allergic reaction. Once I said something, the nurses quickly stopped the machine and gave me more Benadryl. They said I had to get an approval from the doctor before continuing. When the Benadryl kicked in, I got the okay from the doc and continued my infusion. I watched a couple of movies and listened to a book. Once it was complete, I headed home and I had a total range of excitement. The steroids made me feel amazing. Then on top of that, I felt free. For nineteen years I had been confined by medicine that had rough side effects and the whole idea of never feeling that again was overwhelming.

It is amazing how different I felt on this new medication. I felt like layers of goo stuck in my body were finally removed. I felt like a new person. One of the side effects of the other medication I was on was depression. I took medication for that to keep it in check, but I did not realize how much that med was affecting my mental space. Switching to this new infusion allowed me to lower my dose of the anti-depressant anxiety med I had taken since the beginning. I just feel more clearheaded with less "brain congestion."

Freedom and independence are what I have now. No longer does MS run my daily life and now I only deal with slight fatigue. When I look back at all that all I have experienced in the last twenty years, I am shocked by how far I have come and how truly strong I am.

I got to be a part of the National Multiple Sclerosis Society MS Awareness Campaign in 2017 and it was one of the most powerful experiences of my MS journey. To be interviewed exclusively in my own home about my MS story was an incredible feeling. Going to a photoshoot with a few others in the campaign was pretty cool, too. I got to see my good friend Jim

Fairchild being photographed while holding a picture of his daughters, who mean the world to him. Walking in and seeing him getting photographed was so powerful for me and I teared up. I got to meet a couple of other people who were in the campaign and we were instantly bonded for life. The way they edited each person's story was so beautifully done. They truly captured the diversity of MS and the strength all of us who live with MS have. This campaign was seen by hundreds of thousands of people and I really felt like finally my story got to be shared with the world. I managed to push through all the bullshit that comes with living with MS and fight to become who I am on this day. Watching each one of those videos showed me that as powerful as our voices are individually, collectively we are so much louder.

After doing the campaign, I was able to speak at the NMSS Gala Portland 2018, where they played my video for everyone. Then I stood up and gave a speech. My speech was full of emotion, inspiration, and the power of positivity. It was a little daunting to be standing in front of this audience after they had just heard a summary of my story and speak, but I did it successfully. I brought all of the Portland people in the campaign on stage with me and we got a standing ovation. Such a powerful moment to be a part of. Every person in that room was/is affected by MS in some way and they really let us know how incredible we all are. The energy in the room was amazing and full of positive energy. I was approached by a few people telling me how great my speech was. I have been refining my story for over twenty years and it continues to grow and change.

I will continue to reach people through my story and let people see another side of living with MS. I reflect back in awe at how I created this amazing, wonderful life that I lead. My blessed perspective is sacred and I wouldn't change any of it because it made me who I am today.

Journal Entries: 2016

3/7/16

High heels are a crazy invention. Why do women feel the need to be taller or sexier? I was never a huge fan of heels, especially once the MS took over. Not a huge loss for me, being a t-shirt and jeans kind of girl. I am not so into fashion or style. I express myself through all my ink. Although, when there are nice events when I have to dress up, like weddings, I am reminded that I have to wear flats always. Being five feet tall, I can't get those extra inches in heels and look more attractive. Why is that? Why do women feel that makes them look more attractive?

Being able to enlighten people on airplane rides always feels great. Every time I fly with Hatchet people will ask what he does for me. When I tell them I have MS they often say sorry. That is the worst response. I say, I am not. It has made me who I am. I tell them Hatchet has made my life easier. People didn't see me as a drunk, they actually saw me as disabled. On flights, I often had incred-

ible conversations with the person sitting next to me or the stewardess. I found that I really touched people when I talked to them. I really brought the realness of living with a chronic illness to people who never ever thought about it.

8/7/16

Progress, motivation, determination and motion.

Moving forward with so much behind me and slowly, climbing toward the light of center.

Living in the moment, in the present is important and wise. Reflecting on past, sharing the future and being

here, now

present and aware.

Appreciative of what is and thankful for this gift of perspective so young. My perspective is unique and lucky. Thankful for all I am, all I can do and all I will.

Kindness, love, laughter, attitude.

9/10/16

I had minor oral surgery and had to stop smoking for it. I have smoked since I was sixteen, with a year and a half free in 2006. This wasn't because I wanted to, and it was very hard. Even after my diagnosis in 1998, my neurologist said, "The MS isn't gonna kill you, but those cigarettes will." I still continued to smoke. In the beginning I thought, what was the likelihood of me getting diagnosed with another disease? and kept smoking. Smoking has been my crutch through it all. It gave me a way to step away and gave me my own private time.

It has been four days and I hate it. I miss it. I want it so bad, but I know I will not heal properly if I smoke. I am wearing a nicotine patch, but I am greatly wanting that oral fix. I don't know if I will go back or if I can manage to stay strong. I hate it. It is amazing to think of all that I have overcome in the past with the MS. I feel like this is almost bigger then the MS stuff. It is more of a mental battle than all the MS stuff was. The injections, the fear, the walking, the seeing, the heat, the stairs, the questioning. With the MS stuff I didn't feel like I had a choice. I know if I can beat this it would be the biggest thing, but I don't know if I am ready to say goodbye to it or not. I still have ten more days of this and maybe I will feel differently in five days, but as of now I want to smoke. I will smoke more cannabis, which is helping me, but I do feel like something big is missing. I just need to bitch a little. I miss eating food.

10/6/16

Starting a new page in life, trying to find something to be as passionate about as music. I have yet to find what I am looking for. I just turned forty years old and have battled MS for close to twenty years. My passion was and always will be music, but for the last twenty years I have been starved of the pureness of creation of sound other than the two seconds of transitioning, mixing two pieces of music together, nothing compares to playing an instrument and having those vibrations come through your soul.

I am forever trying to find something to do that. I always think everything is too difficult. I just got a mandolin to try and learn something new. Maybe eventually I will be able to get those feelings again through a new instrument. I know practice is key and I give up too quick. Playing music came naturally to me and I learned easily when I was a child. Now, at forty, I have to find those skills again. I will play right now.

Journal Entries: 2017

1/20/17

This new phase of life is a different kind of challenge. I am learning to get out more and interact with people in 3D. I still find it more comfortable to stay home and be alone. This is slowly breaking, but I think I will always feel more comfortable at home, alone. I don't know why I think it is a problem. I enjoy my alone time. I like not having to worry about someone else. At the same time, it would be nice to be able to spend that time with someone who cares about me. Again, patience.

I can now take a couple sips out of a glass using my left hand. I can only do a couple before my tremor starts reacting. The importance of the fact that I can take a couple sips without spilling is overwhelmingly awesome. I have learned my limits and where I have to draw a line through many years of finding that line. It is the little things. I can now use my hand. Now I can tie my shoes. Now I can use two hands to brush my teeth and wash my face. I can now run up and down the stairs. I can now change a light bulb. I can now sit with myself in peace without so much chatter in my head. Only through all of these challenges did I get to the point in my life where I am confident, secure and hopeful. Without all the challenges I faced, I would not be who I am. I have such compassion for people going through challenges they cannot control.

4/21/17

Progress, motivation, determination and motion.

Moving forward with so much behind me and slowing, climbing toward the light of center.

Living in the moment, in the present, is important and wise. Reflecting on the past, sharing the future and being here. Now.

Present and aware.

CHAPTER 9

REFLECTION

*T*his new phase of life is a different kind of challenge. I have such compassion for people going through challenges they cannot control. When I think of all the people I know or have known with progressive MS, whose progression isn't slowed down by drugs, that's what pushes me forward. Because I have beaten a beast, I have gone through enough to learn to push forward even more for all those who can't. I feel so grateful to have regained so much of what I've lost, yet I can't change other people's disease progression. What I can do is bring awareness to the rest of the world about what is often an invisible disease. When I was diagnosed, there were only three drugs available to slow MS's progression. I am ecstatic to say that now there are fifteen drugs to slow the progression of the disease. From what I've seen through the years, there will be a cure in the near future. I couldn't say that for at least ten years, but now, after seeing all the research that's been done and that is happening now, I feel like we will one day live in a world free of MS. It is time for all the able-bodied people in this world to have a new perspective and take a look at what others experience on a daily basis and how they might be able to benefit from help.

What can we do for these people that have no benefit from these medications? It's being done. Those scientists and researchers are figuring out more and more about MS. What they knew sixteen years ago and what they know now blows my mind. After watching my support group develop, and seeing all the people come through with different symptoms, different progressions, and different attitudes, the wide variety of MS is undeniably crazy. Watching what everybody has to deal with symptom-wise as well as in life shows you how strong MS can make you. I think without going through what I went through, I wouldn't be so strong.

The research happening right now is mind-blowing. Not only are they discovering new treatments for those with PPMS and SPMS, they are figuring out how to regenerate the myelin that is damaged. In October of 2018, I was able to go to Oregon Health & Science University and see some of the research they are doing with zebra fish. Zebra fish have an incredible process of myelination. Studying these fish can lead to developing new medications, not just to slow the progression of the disease, but to regenerate what is not there when you have MS. There is so much research going on with new medications and new possibilities. This is a good time to be diagnosed because of all the therapies available and the new ones around the corner. There are more studies available about the power of Eastern Medicine and MS. No stress, lots of sleep, exercise, cannabis, and acupuncture might be the main reasons I am doing as well as I am.

The understanding of the variety and diversity of MS is very important. Because no two people are the same with MS, treatments don't work for everyone and more often than not, patients have to go through the whirlwind of switching medications. I have seen people who have tried five to seven different medications, all with the goal to slow progression, with none working. Fortunately, now there are many different options.

My original neurologist said I needed to get on meds right away because of the progression process. I got on Avonex a month after being diagnosed. I was always amazed by the people who didn't go on any meds. They thought they could control their MS with diet, lifestyle, herbs, and alternative meds. Personally, that scared me. I knew how lucky we were to have all these meds because the generation before me did not have anything to slow the progression down. This illness doesn't stop. The only way to control the progression is through these medications. I always felt a little relief knowing I was doing what I should by continuing these injections, as much as I hated them.

I know everything happens for a reason. I know that I am a fighter. I know I am here to teach the world a little bit about difference, disability, acceptance, fear, hope, and happiness. I want people to realize what they have and appreciate everything that it is. For all these years I pushed myself to be stronger, smarter, wiser, and more grateful. What is life through someone else's eyes?

For all the pain, weakness, numbness, tingling, shaking, dizziness, and discomfort, both physically and mentally, I will push myself. I feel so grateful for what I've accomplished. For all the people who can't push anymore, I push even harder. Any accomplishment, no matter how big or small, will be amazing, but I also know the strength that that my pushing gives others. I'm a bright light of hope and I must share with all those who are welcomed into my world.

Over the years I have participated in many MS events. I have done the MS Walk about eight times through the twenty years. In the beginning, I thought it was silly to have a walk for a bunch of disabled people. I was still angry at the world when I thought this. It took a while to get over that anger and I quickly learned that the MS Walk wasn't really about walking, but about togetherness and solidarity. I began to volunteer at the walks instead of actually walking them. One year I managed to do half of the course, but instead of going across the bridge with everyone else, I trucked over to the Saturday Market and perused all the merchandise. I gave myself credit for making it as far as I did and ended up treating myself to some awesome handmade salt and pepper shakers. I then walked back to the start as everyone came pouring back in. I was there to celebrate with everyone and express my joy to be where I was. A few years later, a couple friends and I walked together with my dog and their kids. It was special to see all the fun everyone was having and how much orange there was all around me. At these events I get to meet others who live with MS, as well as the awesome support people in their lives. With all the generous people giving up their time and energy to help someone in need, we will not get stuck. It is all these people that deserve a round of applause for helping people fight their fight and making it easier for those affected to keep living their best lives. No one can do it alone, no matter how strong they think they are. Only through the support of others do we get through the rough times and rejoice in our accomplishments.

Back in 2005 I had the pleasure of hearing Rayn Prior (Richard Prior's daughter) speak to the MS Society. Her speech was enlightening, hearing all her thoughts about watching her father live with MS. Her attitude and perspective were so positive and inspiring. For someone who lives with MS, it was incredible to hear her stories from the outside. She really allowed us to share her experience. This perspective was something I thought little about at the time, but thinking about all the caretakers and family members who can only sit back and watch it happen, I gained a perspective from a different viewpoint. I reflected on my family and friends, who had to feel so defeated because they would watch what was happening, but couldn't change anything. This inspired me to start speaking at events and sharing my story with all who would listen.

In 2007, I was honored by being asked to speak at the NMSS in Fort Worth, Texas, to acknowledge my grandmother, who had donated a lot of money to the society because of me. There I got to stand in front of a room full of unknown people and share my story and put my face out into the room where people actually were listening to me. I think I affected a lot of them, making them think about things they never had thought about. My words were honest and from my soul and I got a standing ovation. That was the first time I felt the power of my voice and the impact I have on people. That speech gave me strength and I knew in that moment that I was put here on Earth for a purpose. I am here to enlighten other people to make them appreciate their lives a little more and be grateful for all that they have. After the speech was over, so many people came up to me, telling me how powerful my speech was and how incredible of a person I was. I felt amazing and had not felt this powerful in many years.

When the support group was founded, my purpose was to give hope, strength, and courage to all those who heard me. There is a constant flow of positivity in the group, and each person has their own story to share. The knowledge and perspective we get from each other is one that could not be found without each other. Because of the success of the group and staying in contact with the MS Society, I reached out to them to find me more ways to speak to others living with MS. I was able to then do more speeches at events like the MS Walk in Portland and the Bike MS pre-launch event. I was then asked to do an interview for the local radio promoting the power of positivity, sharing my story to a larger audience. I was also asked to speak on a local TV station to bring more awareness to MS. These things built me up to writing my book to share my story with the world.

I will always continue to be a bright light in the MS community. I know that I can affect people with my voice and bring a little awareness to others who live with MS or do not. My story is one of strength, determination, and hope that I think all people could gain some insight from.

I am happy to say that I do think they will find a cure soon. I do think people with PPMS (Primary Progressive), SPMS (Secondary Progressive), and RPMS (Relapsing Progressive) will all be free from further progression because of these new medications they are coming out with. I do think they will find a way to repair the myelin damage that has been done. All the research and progress they have made in the last twenty years is mind-blowing to me and I am happy to say that future generations might never have to deal with all the uncertainty, confusion, and fears of living with MS. Being a part of this community has taught me about incredible perseverance from people who have had intense challenges. We are all making a giant movement in eradicating this disease. I look forward to that day. I will constantly be sharing, enlightening, and bringing hope to all those who feel lost in their own battles be it MS, divorce, or death. Everyone has a battle and learning that you are not alone in your struggle makes the fight a little easier. We are stronger together.

When Selma Blair came out to the world in the middle of an MS flare, the world got to finally see what a flare looked like. Each person with MS is different, so this was just one example of what happens, but it really brought awareness and insight for people who knew nothing about MS. The harsh realities of living with MS were finally shown on television. I know that the MS community gave her a standing ovation for actually showing it. No one really knows the struggle unless you live with it, but this gave healthy people a view of life with MS. There are many famous people who live with MS, but are not as vocal about it. Montel Williams was the first famous person I saw who lived with MS and he gave me so much strength and power to keep on fighting. More and more people are coming out about their MS and showing the world what it is like to battle life with this disease. I don't have such a platform to share, but I am constantly allowing other people to see another side of life. Pretty much every Lyft/Uber ride I have I get to enlighten someone about the life I have led and how my MS has made me who I am today. There is nothing better for me than hearing how grateful they are that they got to pick me up and get a little education on MS and a perspective they had never thought about before.

When I look back over the years, I am in a little disbelief over what I have accomplished. I knew that if I kept pushing, I would see another side of life with MS. I have constantly challenged myself physically and mentally to be free from what I once knew. I feel so honored to live this life where I get the opportunity to enlighten others with the wisdom that the MS has given me. I would never be where I am now without all the struggles, doubts, fears, and triumphs I have experienced. I am happy to say I live with MS, but it doesn't rule my life like it once did. Creating a safe place for people to bitch and moan and celebrate with others who can related to your struggles is really where the power is. No longer feeling alone and being overjoyed to spread my experience with as many people who want to listen has given me a perspective on life that is truly special. I have a gift of words to give others some courage and fortitude to move forward in their lives.

People need to know they are not alone in their battles. Each person who lives with a chronic illness is constantly looking for a cure, but in the meantime we can find ways to live our best lives possible. Our stories need to be shared to help more people through difficult times. We are stronger together with all the support from each other and everyone who supports us.

I am giving people a little more hope in the time of darkness. It has been my mission these last ten years to show the power we have as individuals to make a difference in the world. I look forward to the day when I can say I used to have MS, but it never had me. With the almost one million people who live with MS, together our voices are stronger and more powerful. We will continue to live our best lives and work to create a world without MS.

Journal Entries: 2018

6/25/18

When I look back at all I have accomplished through the years of living with MS I can actually say I am proud of myself. Why is it so hard for me to see the accomplishments and give myself credit? I often compare myself to others and see the things they have that I don't. I try to shift those thoughts to see myself in a different light. Sure, I might not be married or have children or a typical career, but I have gained so much wisdom about living a quality life and seeing beyond the struggles. I climbed out of a dark, deep hole and only now can I look back and say I did a damn good job. I could have thrown up my hands and said I was done, but instead I kept reaching for the top. I have to remind myself constantly how truly strong and capable I am. The difficulties I experienced in daily life for so many years no longer lay so heavy on me. I did crawl out of the hole I was in and now am only searching for the best quality life I can have. The tapes that I had played have been recorded over and I have a new narrative reminding myself of the strength it took to get to where I am and that I did push through all of that bullshit.

Journal Entries: 2019

3/3/19

I am here at the MSPPC19 (National Multiple Sclerosis Society Public Policy Conference) and I am feeling so empowered. Being around all these fellow activists from around the country is such a special treat. I have already met some amazing people. I feel like my life is better than ever. I couldn't be more joyous and grateful for the life I have and for all the shit I went through. Everything has brought me to this point and I am so grateful for all of the struggles because they have brought me to this point. I think I was put here on Earth to be doing exactly what I am doing. Tomorrow we go to Capitol Hill. This afternoon we are creating our HOW, WOW, NOW statements. There is so much information about stuff I rarely think about but is so important to the MS community. When I look around at all these people, I see what amazing, incredible people we all are. The struggle is real, but all the strength and courage gained from those struggles makes or breaks them. This has to be one of the coolest things I have been a part of in my twenty-plus year MS journey. I have not felt this amazing about myself ever. I feel so honored to be a part of this and to get to share part of my story on the Hill.

ABOUT THE AUTHOR

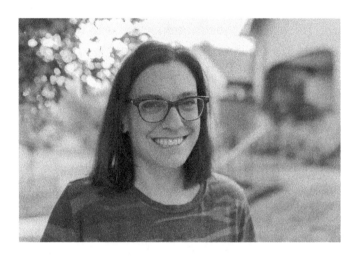

*I*n October 1977, Chloe shocked her mother by coming into the world two and a half months early. Her first two and a half months of life were spent in the hospital, monitoring her health. She grew up in St. Louis, Missouri and spent most of her summers in Colorado. From an early age, Chloe had an interest in music and the outdoors.

She started playing the piano at age five and continued until age twenty. In second grade she took up the cello and played in the orchestra throughout high school. She also played soccer from age six through high school.

At age twenty, Chloe was diagnosed with Multiple Sclerosis and everything she knew of her future was questioned. She was no longer able to do everything that had defined her as a child and a teen. Questions, fears, and uncertainties arose in her head.

Being a musician and now having little use of her left arm, the cello was no longer her musical outlet and she had to find a new way to create music. She started DJing in high school with a few friends who all went in on equipment together. After a few years of processing her diagnosis, she decided to whip out the turntables again to be able to feel the music again. This gave her the feeling she was missing and gave her joy again in her life.

It took many years to adjust to this new life experience. Feeling so alone, she knew there were others out there having similar feelings and experiences and she wanted to find them.

In 2005, she and another woman started a support group for people aged twenty-five and under. Being young and getting hit with disease can be quite brutal. There were others like her out there and they needed to come together.

The group went from twenty-five and unders, to thirty and unders, then became forty-ish and unders. After twelve years, the group changed its name to MS Happy Hour. They meet at a restaurant with a private room just for them, and it is accessible for all. This group gives all who come a little hope and strength for their future. Meeting others who can relate to the struggles, battles, and triumphs really gives people a connection that they need to feel less alone.

Through Chloe's over twenty years of experience in dealing with MS, she has found the power of positive thinking to be crucial to healing and acceptance. Discovering the power of exercise and neuroplasticity has gotten her to where she is today. Working with a personal trainer for the last ten years, she has carved new pathways in her brain and does things now that she once thought were impossible. Her persistence and dedication to her body have allowed this change.

Chloe now speaks to audiences about her experience. She has woken up a lot of people with appreciation of what they have and not what they don't. She speaks of positivity, attitude, and determination.

She was put here on Earth to share her blessed perspective on life with others. Only through struggles and difficulties can a person gain the strength needed to keep on pushing forward. Having others around who can relate to our struggles and accomplishments gives us connection and hope. Together, we are stronger.

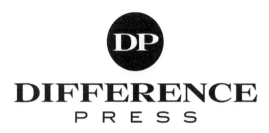

About Difference Press

*D*ifference Press is the exclusive publishing arm of The Author Incubator, an educational company for entrepreneurs – including life coaches, healers, consultants, and community leaders – looking for a comprehensive solution to get their books written, published, and promoted. Its founder, Dr. Angela Lauria, has been bringing to life the literary ventures of hundreds of authors-in-transformation since 1994.

A boutique-style self-publishing service for clients of The Author Incubator, Difference Press boasts a fair and easy-to-understand profit structure, low-priced author copies, and author-friendly contract terms. Most importantly, all of our #incubatedauthors maintain ownership of their copyright at all times.

Let's Start a Movement with Your Message

In a market where hundreds of thousands of books are published every year and are never heard from again, The Author Incubator is different. Not only do all Difference Press books reach Amazon bestseller status, but all of our authors are actively changing lives and making a difference.

Since launching in 2013, we've served over 500 authors who came to us with an idea for a book and were able to write it and get it self-published in less than 6 months. In addition, more than 100 of those books were picked up by traditional publishers and are now available in book stores. We do this by selecting the highest quality and highest potential applicants for our future programs.

Our program doesn't only teach you how to write a book – our team of coaches, developmental editors, copy editors, art directors, and marketing experts incubate you from having a book idea to being a published, bestselling author, ensuring that the book you create can actually make a difference in the world. Then we give you the training you need to use your book to make the difference in the world, or to create a business out of serving your readers.

Are You Ready to Make a Difference?

You've seen other people make a difference with a book. Now it's your turn. If you are ready to stop watching and start taking massive action, go to **http://theauthorincubator.com/apply/**.

"Yes, I'm ready!"

Other Books by Difference Press

Fearful to Fabulous: Unlock Your Power, Move on, and Thrive after Midlife Divorce by Fiona Eckersley

No More Fatigue: A Guide to Increase Energy and Productivity in Everything You Do by Dr. Yani Feliciano

Make Your Own Money Again: Shine Your Light with Purpose and Balance by Charlotte Friborg

Dying To Be Thin: Tools for Battling The Bulimia Beast by Noelle Gilbert RN

Digestive Reset: Fix Your Hormones and Digestion by Balancing Your Gut Microbiome and Adrenals by Inna Lukyanovsky PharmD

Surviving the High School Years with Your Sanity Intact: A Guide for Moms of Out-of-Control Teens by Lisa Gay Nichols

The Profitable & Stress-Free Eye Doctor: The Step-by-Step Guide to Grow a Successful Ortho-K Specialty Business by Dr. Connie Vuong

What You Need to Know to Lead a Marriage Support Group: The Guide to Develop Unity in Marriage by Angela and Chris Yousey

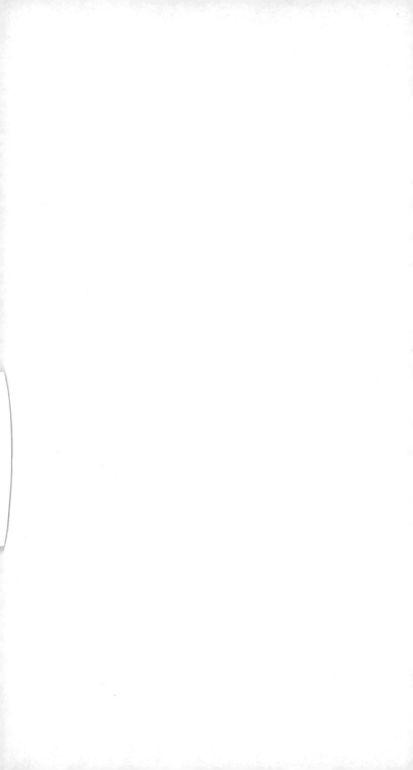